HEIDI MORETTI

Cortisol Fix

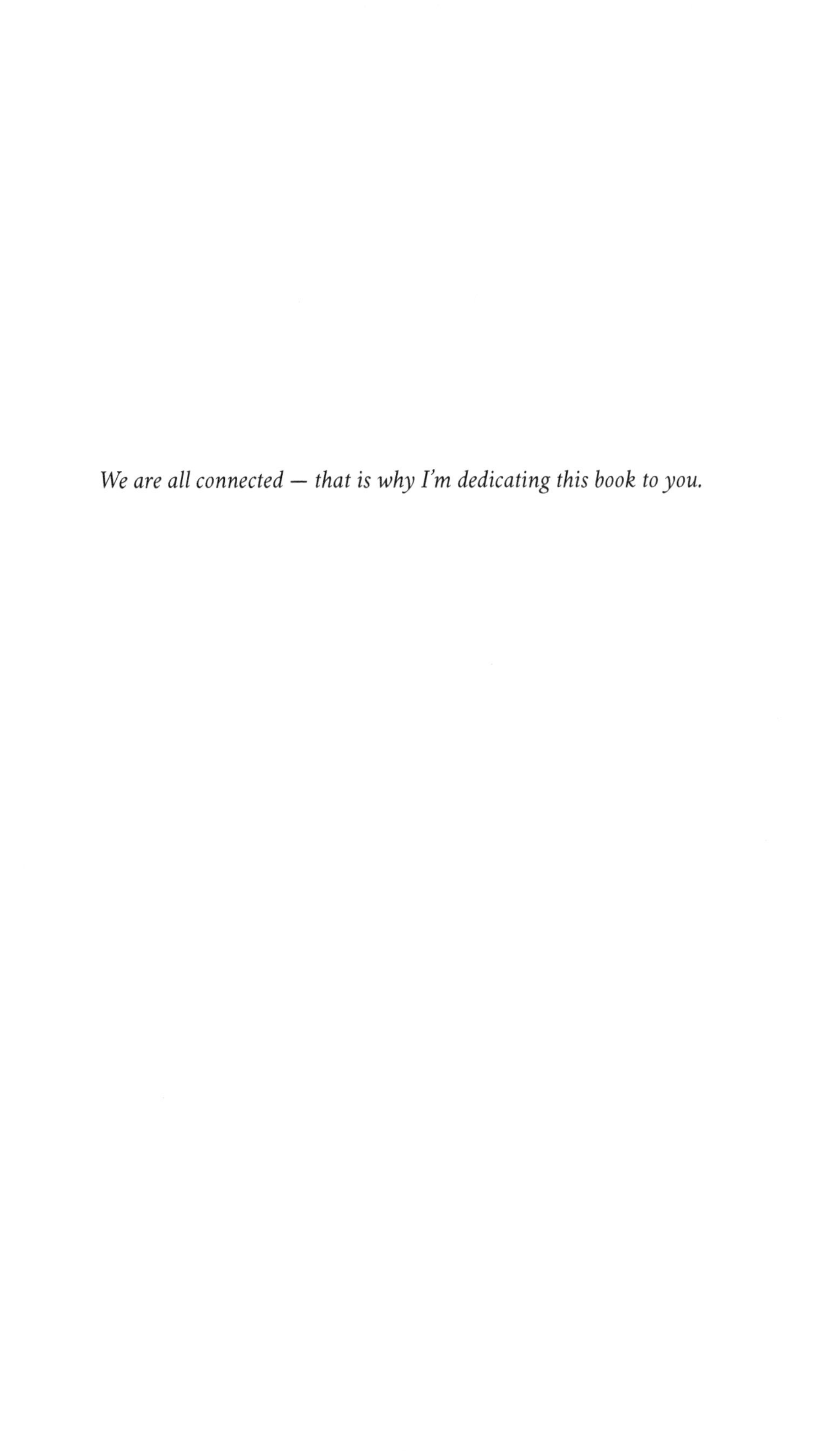

We are all connected — that is why I'm dedicating this book to you.

Normal and optimal are two different things.
You deserve optimal.

Heidi

Contents

Preface

26 years in as a nutrition clinician, researcher, and holistic practitioner, I was called to write this book because **cortisol** is quietly wrecking people's health — and almost no one is talking about it. My training in functional medicine opened my eyes to the possibilities of healing almost everything in a natural way. I've noticed profound and quick changes in my clients' stress and lives when I help them approach their nutrition and lives through the lens of cortisol management.

In each of my clients, I see evidence of stress gone rogue, and often it is the biggest contributor to their health problems and weight gain. Popular weight-loss drugs can't touch this kind of weight gain at its root cause. Stressed-out people are often disappointed with medication management — the medications can further worsen cortisol due to resulting low nutrient stores in the body. It is also clear that the current medical model isn't equipped to deal with these problems. That doesn't mean that things are hopeless; there is a ton of hope, research, and resources for managing cortisol. You will learn a whole lot more about these nutrients and how they help reduce cortisol throughout this book.

I've spent my whole career immersed in the National Library of Medicine, which means that I've learned adept ways to find research. This research often gets overlooked due to the powerful forces of profit-driven companies. You have to know what you are looking for to find it. For example, you have to know that magnesium is depleted by cortisol to find it in the research files. Most doctors have minimal-to-no training in nutrients, so how would they know how to look for this information? They don't. I'm not demeaning the value of doctors, but they know what they know, and it isn't nutrition, for the most part. Unless they specifically seek out this research, doctors will never find it. The medical journals that land on their desks are often highly influenced by the pharmaceutical industry, making it even harder to find unbiased information about stress and cortisol.

Key insight

Here is something your doctor almost certainly hasn't told you: the **stress hormone** your body releases to fight inflammation will, if it stays elevated long enough, cause *more* inflammation.[1] Not less. More.

For all of these reasons, I've been called to write books about natural healing — because I know that this information is not readily available to your doctor or to anyone who isn't willing to spend countless hours seeking out nutritional information in research journals. This is my passion, so I need to share it with you, or else I am not honoring my calling as a healer. It is why I wrote my previous books as well. I wrote *Period Fix* to help women of all ages deal with hormonal issues that are marginalized. I wrote *Gut Fix* because at least 40 percent of people are dealing with gut issues that the current medical model is largely failing.

Addressing the root causes of cortisol imbalances

There are many ways to manage cortisol if you are willing to keep an open mind and use alternative strategies to deal with too much stress. And I bet that's why you are reading this book — to get lasting help that improves your life for the better. I'm excited to help you out on your journey.

Cortisol is the hormone that deals with stress. Its role is to act as a messenger in the body. This messenger can destroy your health. In today's world, it is almost impossible to escape imbalances in this stress hormone. Cortisol imbalance starts with our fast-paced world. This is because our stressful lives overtax the ability of our body to deal with stress in the natural ebb and flow of cortisol. Parenting, taking on caregiver roles, dealing with a lifetime of trauma, traffic, social media, doom-scrolling, and more all take their toll. Unexplained, nagging stress can also seem to come out of nowhere but is often related to our diets and our **gut health**. Food these days is often on the go because people are so busy "doing it all," and these foods are most often highly processed — which ramps up cortisol further. Many people get multiple coffees a day to manage their stress-related fatigue, which drives cortisol even further up. At night, sleep can be poor due to all of these factors, and a lack of restorative sleep causes the cortisol response to worsen. Sound familiar at all? To most people, these scenarios are daily occurrences. Cortisol continues its spiral in our bodies, day in and day out, with little relief.

Here's the kicker: the longer that people have elevated cortisol, the worse the vicious cycle becomes. Long-term stress creates a vicious cycle of stress, poor sleep, an unhealthy gut, nutrient depletion, and out-of-control food cravings. Repeat. It's a stressful world out there, and it shows on your waistline, on your face, in your brain, in your gut, and in your mood. Your whole body suffers from long-term, low-grade, high cortisol.

The root causes of this are apparent, and the solutions to this stress should address its root causes. These root causes for excess cortisol are nutritional imbalances, sleep issues, gut issues, lifestyle factors, work issues, care-giving, trauma, and/or lack of social support.

Cortisol robs the body of nutrients, so a simple way to help reduce cortisol is by replacing those nutrients. I will spend a whole chapter on this, and subsequent chapters on natural approaches to gut health, meal preparation, time-tested natural medicine for cortisol management, exercise, and more.

What this book is and isn't

In this book, I will give you an overview of the causes of cortisol imbalances, the nutritional ways to help with building blocks of hormones and hormone signaling, herbs and natural healing options that dampen cortisol, relaxing exercises, and some simple ways to get more social support. I will also explain other tools that help my clients. But it is always important to seek a multi-pronged approach — therapy and medication management as needed. These should be done under the supervision of your medical provider. And it goes without saying that this book is not meant to be a substitute for seeking out medical care. Rather, it is a starting point to have open conversations with your healthcare team about appropriate options for you as an individual. That said, some healthcare providers can be very closed-minded about natural remedies. You always have the right to seek out second opinions. To find providers that are trained in holistic approaches, I suggest that you find practitioners who are trained in **functional medicine** or highly skilled naturopaths.

In the next chapter, I will discuss how cortisol works, the interplay of cortisol and the whole body, and an introduction to cortisol, food, and nutrients.

Acknowledgments

I'm thankful for Jenn Chau, Kobe Chau, Erna Wenus, Clark Patton, and all the unsung healers out there for motivating me to write this book and for helping people overcome their stress and trauma.

1

Chapter 1

CORTISOL 101 — ITS WIDESPREAD EFFECTS ON YOUR HEALTH

Loving and caring for yourself is a powerful gift to the world. By helping to understand what cortisol is and what it does, you can more easily care for yourself and others. In this chapter, you will learn the basics of cortisol and its connections to whole-body health, food impacts on cortisol, the impacts of chronic stress, and testing cortisol. You will also learn how to identify symptoms of too much stress signaling in your body.

Cortisol, the party crasher

Picture a party. Everything's going well — good music, good food, everyone behaving themselves. Then one guy shows up. Let's call him Cort.

Cort is fine in small doses. Cort is actually *useful* in small doses — he's the one who notices when something's wrong, sounds the alarm, gets everyone moving. But Cort has been hitting the open bar since 2009, and at this point he's not reading the room. He's lecturing strangers about their life choices. He's knocked something off a shelf. He's somehow simultaneously exhausted and furious, and he has strong opinions about the thermostat.

That's chronic cortisol. Not the helpful alarm signal your body was designed to use occasionally — but the version that never got the memo that the emergency is over.

The party guests Cort has been bullying? Those are your other hormones. **Ghrelin**, **leptin**, **GLP-1**, estrogen, thyroid hormone, insulin — all of them trying to do their jobs while Cort elbows through the crowd knocking drinks out of people's hands. An unhealthy **gut microbiome** makes this worse, because your gut is essentially the venue management — responsible for keeping Cort's behavior in check — and if the venue is a mess, nobody's getting Cort under control.

The good news: Cort can be managed. And it's more straightforward than you'd think. That's what this chapter — and this book — is here to show you.

A simplified look at cortisol and stress

Think of cortisol as a text message. Your body sends it to your tissues when something needs attention: danger nearby, raise blood pressure, mobilize energy, focus up. Useful! Necessary! Great in the moment.

The problem isn't the text. The problem is when the texts never stop.

Imagine your phone buzzing every four minutes, all day, every day, for years. At some point your brain stops registering the notifications. You become numb to them. Your body does the same thing with cortisol — a phenomenon called **cortisol resistance**, which we'll get into shortly, and which explains why chronically stressed people often feel simultaneously wired and utterly flattened.[1] The alarm keeps going off. Nothing responds to it anymore. Another reason you might want to manage your cortisol levels is that too much cortisol is related to early aging.[3]

Sustained high cortisol isn't just exhausting — it's a genuine health hazard. We're talking elevated risk of heart disease, diabetes, depression, high blood pressure, stroke, and accelerated aging.[1,2] Not as a distant theoretical possibility, but as documented outcomes of the same cortisol overload that millions of people are walking around with right now, largely unaddressed, because conventional medicine doesn't have a prescription for it.

One clarification worth making early: cortisol isn't the absolute villain here. Exercise raises cortisol — and exercise is obviously good for you in doses. The spike from a hard workout is followed by a meaningful drop, and your body comes out better balanced than before. That's cortisol working correctly. The problem is chronic elevation without recovery. Cort at the party for one night is fine. Cort who has moved into your spare bedroom is a different situation entirely.

When you have high cortisol levels, you are stressed — but that's not all. This **fight or flight** hormone gets you going and motivates you. Cortisol text messages have other important functions, including immune function, glucose management, inflammation regulation, digestive function, and even metabolism of nutrients.[2]

Cortisol's quieter cousin: cortisone

Here's something most people have never heard of: cortisone — not the injection your orthopedist talks about, but the naturally occurring version your body makes from cortisol.

If cortisol is the loud, reactive version of your stress response, **cortisone** is the calmer, gentler metabolite your body converts it into once the emergency has passed. Think of cortisol as the fire alarm and cortisone as the all-clear signal. For ideal health, you want your body converting cortisol to cortisone efficiently — keeping the ratio low, keeping the alarm from ringing indefinitely.

Your liver, gut, kidneys, and fat tissue all handle this conversion.[4,5] Which means that if any of those systems are struggling — **fatty liver disease**, gut inflammation, kidney issues — the conversion slows down, cortisol stays elevated longer than it should, and Cort keeps partying while everyone else is trying to sleep.

Microplastics, it turns out, directly impair this conversion.[6] Which is one more excellent reason to stop microwaving food in plastic containers, stop drinking from plastic bottles left in hot cars, and generally treat plastic contact with your food as the low-grade health hazard it increasingly appears to be. Fresh produce supports the conversion.[7] **Microplastics** undermine it. Nature continues to be right about things.

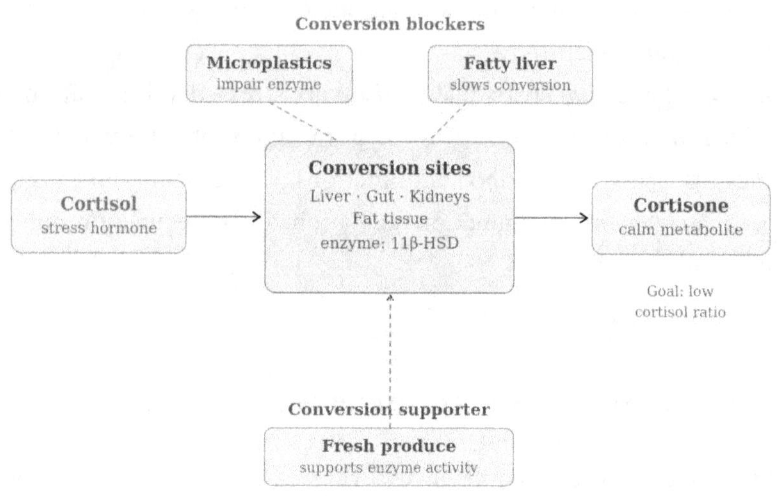

Diagram 1: Cortisol-to-cortisone conversion pathway — showing liver, gut, kidneys, and fat tissue as conversion sites; microplastics and fatty liver as conversion blockers; fresh produce as a conversion supporter.

The other good news is that cortisol text excess is fixable and can be simple, both in the short term and long term. Here's a great short-term example of a Cortisol Fix. Think about a time when you had a really wholesome meal and it made you feel great, both physically and mentally. For me, a good example of this would be a homemade stew or a fresh salmon salad followed by a nice cup of herbal tea. What might this meal be for you? These nutritious meals can dampen down cortisol text message response to appropriate levels. Imagine if you also incorporated targeted nutritional supplements, herbs, exercise, and stress management tools that help dampen cortisol for a longer period of time. You would be in a much better state of physical and mental health.

By the way, there are essentially no prescription medications that address cortisol messaging effectively for chronically elevated stress levels, so it is up to you to do the work on your nutrition and health. That is the point of this book — to help get you on the right path. While the exception to this is Cushing's disease, a rare disease of excess cortisol due to pituitary issues or prescription cortisol medications, most people's cortisol is fixable.

Everything is connected

Your body is not a collection of separate systems that occasionally run into each other in the hallway. It is one deeply interconnected web, where a disturbance in one corner sends ripples through everything else.

Here's a simple illustration. You eat a piece of cake. Delicious, completely worth it, no regrets. But in your gut, the sugar and the absence of any useful nutrients triggers a small alarm.[8] Your gut bacteria — disrupted, underfed, unimpressed — send a distress signal up to your brain. Your brain, receiving what it interprets as a threat signal, responds by dispatching inflammatory chemicals and cortisol. You are now mildly stressed because of cake. This is not a metaphor. This is your actual physiology.

Eat wild salmon with roasted vegetables and sauerkraut instead, and your gut sends an entirely different signal. Happy bacteria, happy brain, balanced hormones, lower cortisol. The meal you eat for lunch is having a conversation with your stress hormones whether you're aware of it or not.

And cortisol doesn't stay in its lane. When it's chronically elevated, it drags every other hormone into the chaos:

- **Thyroid hormone** goes haywire, causing bowel changes, altered gut bacteria, and anxiety.
- **Estrogen** climbs — driven by both gut imbalances and cortisol excess — leading to a condition called **estrogen dominance**, which raises breast cancer risk and causes men to develop female-pattern weight gain. (Yes, really.)
- **Testosterone** and **progesterone** drop, because cortisol is metabolically upstream of both and will cannibalize their building blocks without a second thought.

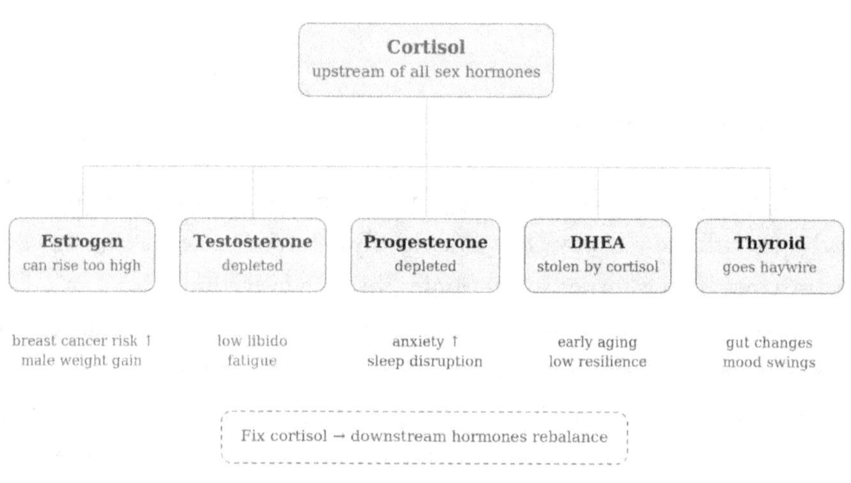

Diagram 2: Hormone hierarchy — cortisol upstream of estrogen, testosterone, progesterone, and DHEA. Arrows showing how chronic cortisol elevation disrupts each downstream hormone.

The hormonal system, in other words, is only as stable as its most disruptive member. And right now, for most people, that member is Cort — still at the party, still not going home, loudly explaining to your thyroid why it's doing everything wrong.

The fix is not as complicated as all this sounds. Getting your gut healthy and your nutrition dialed in tends to bring Cort into line faster than almost anything else. That's the thread running through this entire book, and we'll pull on it from every direction.

Your body's own words

Here is a brief story, written by your body, to demonstrate how everything is connected:

Cortisol: "Hi, I'm cortisol. I'm supposed to be neutralized here, in the gut."

Gut: "Nope, can't do it — you ate too much sugar and you don't have enough probiotics and nutrients to neutralize that cortisol."

Cortisol: "Fine, we'll go back into the bloodstream and be 'extra.' We'll see how you like that, body!"

Body: "Why am I gaining weight, having mood swings, bloating, acne, and insomnia?"

Gut: "Get me back on track and then we can help fix that cortisol, which is causing most of your problems."

Cortisol: "Fine, I'll just raise blood sugar then."

Gut: "I literally cannot with you right now."

Trauma and cortisol connections to nutrition

Cortisol and mental health are tightly connected. The impact of traumatic experiences extends far beyond psychological well-being. A growing body of research shows a profound connection between trauma, cortisol, and the state of gut health and nutrition. The interplay between our brain and gut is a complex system but is incredibly important.8 This system plays a vital role in our response to stress, so optimizing gut health through nutrition can help you manage your response to stress.

There's an actual communication highway running between your brain and your gut called the **gut-brain axis**. It's a two-way system — your brain talks to your gut, your gut talks back — and it uses three different languages simultaneously: nerve signals, hormones, and immune messengers. The main road is the **vagus nerve**, a remarkable piece of biological infrastructure that connects your brain stem directly to your digestive tract, heart, and lungs. Think of it as the interstate between your emotions and your digestion. When one end is in chaos, the other knows about it immediately.

Here's the part that surprises most people: your gut is not just a passive recipient of stress signals. It's an active participant. Your gut houses millions of neurons — enough that scientists have taken to calling it the "second brain" — and produces roughly 95% of your body's **serotonin**. Not your brain. Your gut. The organ you've been ignoring since that questionable burrito in 2019 is manufacturing the majority of your mood-regulating chemistry.

So what happens when trauma or chronic stress enters the picture?

Cortisol floods the system. And cortisol, as we've established, is not a gracious house guest. In the gut specifically, it does four things, none of them helpful:

- Slows or disrupts the muscle movements that keep digestion running smoothly
- Triggers immune changes that inflame the gut lining
- Accelerates nutrient loss — your body literally excretes vitamins and minerals faster under stress
- Knocks your gut bacteria out of balance, which then worsens your stress response, which then worsens your gut bacteria, which then — you see where this is going

The loop is vicious and it's self-reinforcing. But here's the genuinely hopeful part: because the gut-brain axis runs in both directions, healing the gut directly improves your stress response. You don't have to fix your trauma before you fix your gut. You can work from the gut upward — using nutrition, targeted supplements, and the tools in this book — and watch the mental and emotional symptoms start to shift as a result.

That's not wishful thinking. That's the gut-brain axis working in your favor for once. Our gut influences all of our body and mind functions, including digestion, mood, memory, health, and even our response to stress and fear.[18]

Stomach medications: a root cause of cortisol problems?

Let's talk about something that genuinely frustrates me — and should frustrate you too.

One of the most common ways cortisol gut problems get worse isn't the stress itself. It's the medication prescribed to treat the symptoms of the stress. Specifically, **proton pump inhibitors** and other stomach acid drugs — the little pills handed out for heartburn, reflux, and stomach discomfort that have become some of the most prescribed medications in the world.

Here's what the prescription pad doesn't mention:

- These drugs reduce nutrient absorption significantly, depleting the very vitamins and minerals your body needs to regulate cortisol[9,10]
- They disrupt gut bacteria balance, which — as we've just established — directly worsens your stress response[9,10]
- Children taking these medications are more than 2.5 times as likely to develop anxiety and depression.[1]
- Adults taking them face more than double the risk of anxiety and suicidal thoughts[11]

Worth pausing on
A medication routinely prescribed for heartburn is associated with a

twofold increase in suicidal ideation. We can't say with absolute certainty that the drug causes this — correlation isn't causation — but as risk factors go, that one is hard to look away from.[11]

What makes this particularly maddening is that in my 26 years of practice, I have almost never encountered a stomach acid case I couldn't address through nutrition and holistic approaches. Almost never. The root cause of most reflux and heartburn isn't too much stomach acid — it's the wrong foods, imbalanced gut bacteria, and nutrient deficiencies. Fix those, and the symptoms resolve. No prescription required.

If you're currently taking a stomach acid medication, here are three things worth knowing:

1. **Don't stop abruptly without guidance.** Stopping PPIs cold turkey can cause rebound acid surges that feel worse than the original problem. Work with a knowledgeable provider — ideally one trained in functional medicine or nutrition — to wean off gradually while addressing the underlying cause.

2. **Supplement aggressively while you're on them.** If you're not ready to stop yet, or can't, protect yourself. These drugs particularly deplete magnesium, B12, vitamin C, zinc, and iron.[9,10] All of the supplements discussed in Chapter 6 become even more critical if you're taking acid-blocking medications.

3. **Restore your gut bacteria.** Whether you're on stomach acid drugs, have recently finished a course of antibiotics, or both — a quality multi-strain probiotic is non-negotiable. Antibiotics in particular can leave your microbiome so disrupted that cortisol dysregulation, immune dysfunction, and mood issues follow in their wake. Rebuilding takes time and intention. Chapter 8 covers exactly how to do this.

None of this is to say these medications are never necessary. Sometimes they are. But "sometimes necessary" has quietly become "reflexively prescribed to anyone who mentions heartburn," and that gap — between appropriate use and overuse — is where a lot of unnecessary suffering lives.

For a deeper dive into this topic, I cover the full picture in my book *Gut Fix*. But the short version is this: if you're on these medications and wondering why your anxiety, energy, and mood aren't improving despite doing everything else right, this could be a significant piece of the puzzle.

Cortisol damages the gut

Cortisol has been linked to a variety of gut health problems and nutritional problems. Cortisol and trauma cause damage in the gut, often leading to chronic gut disorders. Studies have found a higher prevalence of **IBS** (irritable bowel syndrome) and other gastrointestinal issues among veterans with **PTSD**, but this would also be true of anyone with traumatic stress.[18] Such conditions not only affect our physical health but can also amplify feelings of anxiety and depression, forming a vicious cycle of stress and discomfort.

One of the best parts of my job is that I get to see my clients rapidly experience a reduction in anxiety by simply addressing their gut issues nutritionally and holistically. The solutions don't have to be overly complicated either. Fixing nutritional deficiencies, using safe and effective herbal supplements, and building in simple diet strategies are most often enough to balance cortisol levels.

The link between the gut and stress is not a one-way street. Just as stress can influence gut health, the state of our gut can have a significant impact on mental well-being. Poor gut health can worsen stress and cortisol symptoms. This is true because of the gut's role in producing neurotransmitters like serotonin and melatonin, and the gut's impact on systemic inflammation.[8,18]

Imbalances in gut bacteria can worsen brain function and mood. By doing so, imbalances in gut bacteria also intensify stress symptoms and the body's cortisol response.[8] On the other hand, a healthy gut — promoted by a balanced diet, good nutrition, targeted nutritional supplements, and herbs — can support better mental health and help reduce many cortisol symptoms. I will review a lot of these tips and tricks in Chapter 8.

Symptoms of chronically elevated cortisol

Cortisol text messages in our body can be hard to discern. Stress doesn't always show up in the body in predictable ways. You can experience low levels of any of the following symptoms if your cortisol levels are imbalanced:

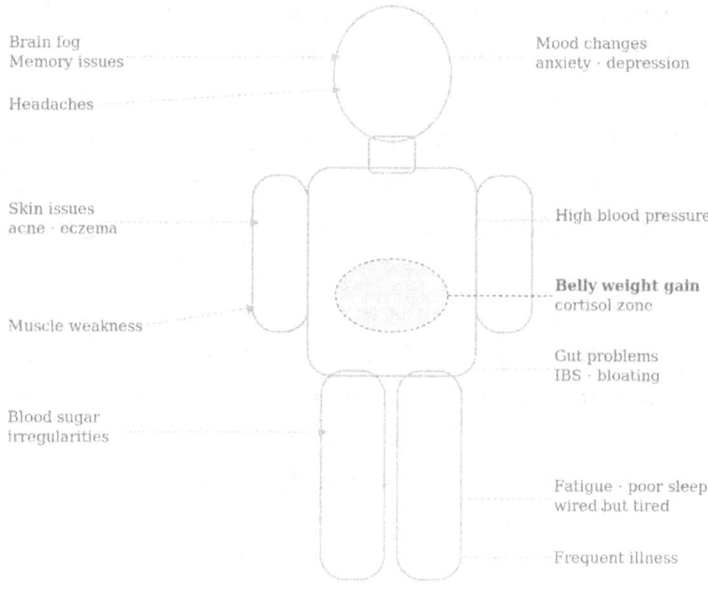

Graphic 1: Body silhouette with symptoms mapped to body regions — brain

fog/memory issues at head; headaches at temples; mood changes at brain; high blood pressure at heart; belly weight gain at abdomen; blood sugar irregularities at pancreas; gut issues at intestines; skin issues at skin layer; muscle weakness at limbs.

- **Fatigue**, particularly feeling "wired but tired"
- **Weight gain**, especially around the abdomen
- **Difficulty sleeping** despite feeling exhausted
- **Frequent illness** or feeling run-down
- **Muscle weakness**
- **Headaches**
- **High blood pressure**
- **Skin issues** like eczema, acne, or slow wound healing
- **Blood sugar irregularities** — there goes Cort again, raiding the snack table
- **Mood changes**: anxiety, irritability, depression, and mood swings
- **Memory difficulties**: difficulty concentrating, brain fog, and memory problems
- **Increased stress and anxiety**: elevated cortisol is linked to heightened stress and anxiety responses

Some people have elements of all of these symptoms every day, making it hard to know what normal should feel like. These types of symptoms also can have many different root causes. The source of your headaches can be food sensitivities, stress, injury, dehydration, and/or lack of nutrients. The beauty is that you can fix the root causes of cortisol imbalances.

It is critical to fix cortisol imbalances at the root. Cortisol steals from other hormones or causes other hormones to be out of balance, as I will discuss next.

The cortisol steal

Just as cortisol disrupts gut balances and nutrient absorption, it is a thief from other hormones. You see, cortisol is metabolically upstream from most other hormones, and if you have too much cortisol, you won't be able to make enough estrogen, testosterone, progesterone, or even **DHEA**.[2] On the other hand, cortisol can cause high levels of hormones such as thyroid hormone and estrogen. Repetitive stress makes the body lean towards survival mode. Cortisol will also make you more likely to get diabetes, in part due to an inappropriate response to insulin caused by stress.[1] Whether you are a woman or a man, this lack of hormonal balance is exceptionally debilitating to your whole body's vital functions. This is part of why people gain weight in their abdomen when they have cortisol imbalance.

Is adrenal fatigue real?

Perched on top of your kidneys are two tiny glands called the adrenals. They're about the size of a walnut. For their size, they do an almost comical amount of work — pumping out cortisol every time life throws something stressful your way, then recovering, then doing it again. They're remarkably good at this, with one catch: they need a moment between rounds. When stressful events arrive faster than the adrenals can recover — which, in modern life, is basically always — things start to go sideways.

This brings us to one of medicine's more entertaining semantic debates: adrenal fatigue.

The conventional medical establishment does not officially recognize **adrenal fatigue** as a real diagnosis. This position is stated with great confidence by people who will then turn around and acknowledge that chronic stress causes fatigue, brain fog, body aches, low libido, caffeine dependence, and a general sense that your get-up-and-go got up and left.[12] The symptoms are real. The suffering is real. The argument is mostly about what to call it.

Here's what's actually happening underneath those symptoms, which may settle the debate more usefully than any naming convention:

Two things tend to be going on simultaneously. First, nutritional depletion — chronic cortisol elevation burns through iron, vitamin A, magnesium, selenium, and a long list of other nutrients that your stress response literally cannot function without.[2] Second, cortisol resistance — the same phenomenon that gives us insulin resistance, except applied to cortisol.[12] When cortisol stays elevated for long enough, your body's receptors essentially stop listening to it. The signal keeps firing. Nothing responds. You feel simultaneously stressed and completely flat, which is as unpleasant as it sounds.

So if you've brought these symptoms to a doctor and been told that adrenal fatigue isn't real — they're technically correct about the diagnosis and practically unhelpful about your actual situation. The more useful framing is cortisol resistance, which is both well-documented and, crucially, fixable.[12]

Nutritional repletion and holistic approaches can restore cortisol sensitivity over time. Your adrenals are small but they are resilient. Give them the right support and they will absolutely get back to work.

Cortisol resistance due to chronic stress

Chronic stress causes a lot of problems with your health, and one of the reasons this happens is that the body becomes resistant to cortisol. Prolonged cortisol release causes a desensitization. A good comparison of this would be a police officer who deals with stressful situations on a daily basis. His or her body adapts and reacts less to the spike of cortisol that occurs with each stressful situation. But this cortisol resistance is linked to many different diseases like Alzheimer's disease, Parkinson's disease, and depression.[13] Part of the reason that long-term cortisol imbalance causes these diseases is due to the ongoing release of inflammatory compounds due to cortisol.[14] The body tries to adjust to this by making **melatonin**, but ultimately this doesn't work to adequately balance the body.

Progesterone and cortisol

Progesterone is closely connected to cortisol and overall hormonal balance. Low progesterone levels are associated with elevated cortisol and increased anxiety symptoms.[18] This connection is especially relevant for women experiencing perimenopause and menopause, where declining progesterone levels are associated with elevated 24-hour urinary cortisol levels and worsening mood and sleep disturbances.[19] Cort at 3am, causing ruckus in the cabinets. Optimizing progesterone levels under the guidance of a healthcare provider may be an important part of a comprehensive cortisol management plan.[18,19]

I'm stressed! Should I measure my cortisol?

I think that hormonal testing is exceptionally valuable. However, another way to look at it is that if you are stressed all of the time, cortisol will be elevated, so why bother checking it? Testing also won't uncover whether or not you have cortisol resistance. In this situation, I think it's a highly personalized decision. If you are the type of person who likes to see measurable changes, I would recommend checking cortisol levels. But this is where healthcare providers definitely don't agree on the best method of doing so. In my experience, the **DUTCH hormone test** is a great starting point because it checks urinary levels of cortisol at multiple points in the day while also checking other hormones. This test measures many hormones, including cortisol, DHEA, estrogen, progesterone, and testosterone. DHEA itself, as I reviewed in my book *Period Fix*, is a helpful value to know because optimizing it can improve feelings of well-being and dampen stress itself. The DUTCH test is clinically validated as a sensitive and specific marker for hormone levels, including cortisol.[15]

Many people these days are testing a marker of cortisol response called **heart rate variability**. Heart rate variability (HRV) is the variation in the time between heartbeats. The theory is that a person with low stress will have a higher heart rate variability, and people with high stress will have a low heart rate variability. Results from research are unfortunately disappointing in this regard in terms of true cortisol response.[16,17] While I think heart rate variability can be a helpful measure of heart health and mental health, it isn't for everyone. It requires wearing a tech device such as a smartwatch or fitness tracker, which could lead to more time on your device — potentially drawing your attention to stressful media or doom-scrolling.

Regardless of whether you test cortisol or not, addressing stress by healing your gut and using natural, supportive health strategies will get you on the path to healing from excess cortisol. When in doubt, start with your gut and support systems.

References

1 Incollingo Rodriguez AC, et al. Cortisol dysregulation and metabolic syndrome. *Nutrients.* 2022. https://pubmed.ncbi.nlm.nih.gov/35743423/

2 Paragliola RM, et al. Cortisol excess and adrenal insufficiency. *Int J Mol Sci.* 2020. https://pmc.ncbi.nlm.nih.gov/articles/PMC7749606/

3 Epel ES, et al. Accelerated telomere shortening in response to life stress. *Proc Natl Acad Sci USA.* 2004. https://pubmed.ncbi.nlm.nih.gov/19320982/

4 Tomlinson JW, et al. 11beta-hydroxysteroid dehydrogenase type 1. *Endocr Rev.* 2004. https://pmc.ncbi.nlm.nih.gov/articles/PMC4698606/

5 Nixon M, et al. Corticosteroid metabolism. *Curr Opin Pharmacol.* 2006. https://pubmed.ncbi.nlm.nih.gov/16061836/

6 Microplastics and glucocorticoid metabolism. *Sci Total Environ.* 2024. https://www.sciencedirect.com/science/article/pii/S014765132401604X

7 Holt SH, et al. Diet and cortisol metabolism. *Eur J Clin Nutr.* 2023. https://pubmed.ncbi.nlm.nih.gov/23364022/

8 Mayer EA, et al. Gut-brain axis and the microbiota. *J Clin Invest.* 2015.

https://www.ncbi.nlm.nih.gov/pmc/articles/PMC4366209/

9 Proton pump inhibitors and microbiome. *Nutrients.* 2022. https://pmc.ncbi.nlm.nih.gov/articles/PMC9099128/

10 Lombardo L, et al. PPI and bacterial overgrowth. *Dig Dis Sci.* 2010. https://pubmed.ncbi.nlm.nih.gov/16524691/

11 Laudisio A, et al. PPI and neuropsychiatric outcomes. *Sci Rep.* 2022. https://www.nature.com/articles/s41598-022-24244-z

12 Razzoli M, et al. Glucocorticoid receptor resistance. *Front Endocrinol.* 2018. https://pmc.ncbi.nlm.nih.gov/articles/PMC3341031/

13 Cortisol resistance and neurodegeneration. *Brain Res Rev.* 2024. https://pmc.ncbi.nlm.nih.gov/articles/PMC10706127/

14 HPA axis in chronic stress. *Neurosci Biobehav Rev.* 2023. https://pmc.ncbi.nlm.nih.gov/articles/PMC9823716/

15 DUTCH test validation. *Front Endocrinol.* 2021. https://pmc.ncbi.nlm.nih.gov/articles/PMC7962249/

16 Kim HG, et al. HRV and stress biomarkers. *Front Physiol.* 2018. https://pmc.ncbi.nlm.nih.gov/articles/PMC5967249/

17 Koenig J, et al. Limitations of HRV in stress research. *Psychosom Med.* 2021. https://pubmed.ncbi.nlm.nih.gov/33390146/

18 Gut microbiota and stress biomarkers. *Nutrients.* 2021. https://pmc.ncbi.nlm.nih.gov/articles/PMC7744704/

19 Menopause symptoms and elevated 24-hour urinary cortisol levels. *Maturitas.* 2011. https://pubmed.ncbi.nlm.nih.gov/21037488/

2

Chapter 2

BABY, YOU WERE BORN THIS WAY

To understand why cortisol is so hard to escape today, we need to start before birth. Our lives are shaped by it all. Let's explore human growth and development and societal pressures that can make or break the quality of our lives.

Cortisol in childhood is a societal problem

Our stress starts before we are born. This is, in part, because our mothers and fathers often aren't allowed time to care for and nurture themselves well. Parents' resources are ridiculously limited in today's world, especially if they are poor. But our whole society is burdened with trauma as a result, as you will soon learn.[1]

Even in the best of child-raising scenarios, our society sets us up with impossible obstacles. We are all expected to perform better, do more with less, be a perfect parent, care for our own parents or loved ones, and all the while work full-time. Our bodies and minds were not well-adapted to deal with all of this. It is high time that we make changes to our environment so we do not have to constantly adapt to more and more hostility around us.

As humans, we are born helpless. Our brains are so big, but our bodies and minds are undeveloped. We need constant care and nurturing from our mothers, fathers, and community to develop properly. Without this care, we would perish rather quickly. While very cursory protections are in place for caring for our infants, such as 12-week family medical leave laws, many small companies don't have to abide by these rules. And if you haven't noticed, a 12-week-old human baby is still not very well equipped to deal with the world. Rather than having a parent or trusted family member able to watch this infant, we are often relegated to paying for daycare and essentially leaving our young infants to chance. Some people aren't even that lucky. They are forced to rely on very questionable circumstances to raise their babies. These circumstances can lead to outright abuse and create immeasurable societal burdens, as seen in **trans generational trauma**.[1] **PTSD** is an infectious disease that is carried from one generation to the next. These abuses and neglect lead to a lifetime of trauma and stress that can lead to PTSD and difficulties functioning as a productive member of society.

Men and boys aren't immune from trauma either. Sometimes their traumas are worse because they are taught that they aren't allowed to show their emotions. And this sometimes manifests in very ugly ways. They may deal with their own trauma by hating themselves, hating women, abusing women, abusing themselves, and passing on emotional traumas. That's a whole book by itself!

We are not necessarily encouraged, but also not discouraged, to feed our babies subpar baby formula from the get-go. We have to drop our babies off with strangers so that we can work to make ends meet — essentially working day and night without rest. OK, I know what you are thinking. Formula-fed babies are OK, and yes, they are, but this is by no means a close substitute for mothers' milk. I was formula-fed, and I'm writing this book, so it will be OK. But it's not to say that I don't suffer for it health-wise, as do all other formula-fed babies. Our immune systems and whole bodies and minds will never be optimized on corn syrup solid-based, factory-made baby formula.

The wolf pack principle

Think of wolves. They huddle pregnant females in the center of the pack — protected, fed, supported. Meanwhile, we hand new mothers a 12-week leave policy and a casserole. That sense of collective safety is exactly what keeps cortisol in check — and exactly what most of us are missing.

Unlike what our capitalist culture teaches, we are not supposed to do it all. It truly does take a village to raise a child.

We have let our society fall apart by forcing a chin-up, do-it-yourself, be-all-you-can-be mentality — and our cortisol — and our waistlines — show it.

We are designed to be like responsible mammals — to care for each other. But in Westernized/capitalist societies, this all falls to the wayside. Minimal-to-no concessions are made to adapt our work environments to support our health. There are no concessions made to care for our babies once that mere 12 weeks is over. Single women and their children have heartbreaking stories of how their resources are dried up and there is essentially little-to-no support due to policy changes in the United States. Our society depends on raising every child well.

While violence has many causes, a lack of nurturing of our young children is certainly part of this phenomenon. Children who aren't nurtured well are also more likely to end up in the prison system, ultimately costing way more money than they would have cost had they been supported in a holistic way.[1]

Now, think of this concept from the perspective of the baby. They are only 12 weeks old and they don't know why their attentive care is no longer there. Their nurturing is stunted and their basic needs may not be met. Emotionally, this takes a toll for a lifetime. The little baby's brain doesn't know why its needs aren't being met, and they develop traumas — big and small — from the start. And some children face big traumas only to carry them over to the next generation because they don't know how to face their own demons. Not to mention the overt traumas that people experience due to the societal pressure for all women to look like Barbie dolls the second after we deliver a baby.

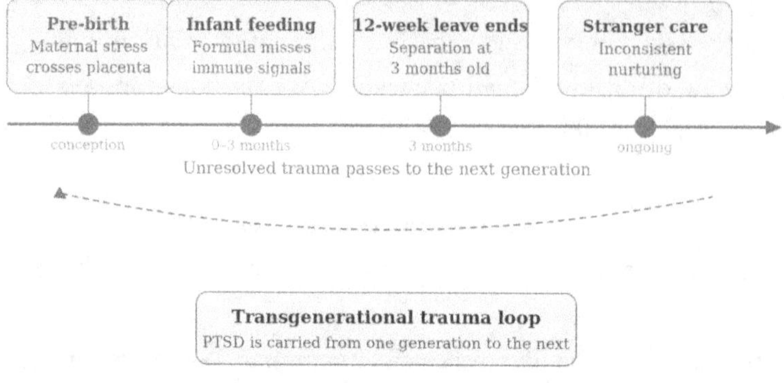

*Graphic 1: Timeline of cortisol stress points from pre-birth through infancy —
showing prenatal maternal stress, formula versus breast milk, daycare separation
at 12 weeks, and the generational trauma loop.*

Societal pressures make our hormones imbalanced

Layer on top of all this the reality of modern eating. When there's no time
to cook — and for most people there genuinely isn't — ultra-processed
convenience food fills the gap. Which means the nutrient deficiencies
driving cortisol imbalance get worse, not better, precisely when life is most
demanding. Nutrient depletion and cortisol dysregulation feed each other
in a loop that's very hard to break from the outside.

Then add phones. Social media. The constant low-grade stimulation that
has colonized not just our own nervous systems but our children's too. Our

hormonal systems were not designed for this level of input, and they are showing the strain — nutritionally, emotionally, and in every chronic disease statistic we have. The violence, the mood disorders, the epidemic of anxiety in people who are technically fine on paper — these are not random. They are the accumulated weight of a thousand small deprivations that start, as we've seen, before birth.[1]

And then, because apparently that wasn't enough, we add body image into the mix.

Women are expected to emerge from childbirth looking like they simply borrowed a baby for nine months and promptly returned it. We're handed impossible standards by social media, contradictory nutrition advice from healthcare providers, and cultural messaging that treats eating as something to be managed rather than enjoyed. Meanwhile — worth stating clearly — cholesterol, which gets relentlessly demonized, is actually essential for infant brain development. The nutrient we've spent decades fearing is one a growing baby genuinely cannot do without.

The result of all this is a society quietly passing its unresolved wounds from one generation to the next. People who weren't nurtured struggle to nurture. People who grew up with disordered relationships with food pass those patterns on. The generational transmission of trauma is not a concept — it is a documented, measurable phenomenon, and it shows up in cortisol levels, gut health, and mental health outcomes across entire family lines.[1]

None of this is inevitable.

I have watched people recover from profound trauma — nutritionally, emotionally, physiologically — using approaches that actually work. Real recovery. Not managed symptoms, but genuine healing. The next section covers the strategies I return to again and again with my clients, so that you have a starting point that doesn't require you to figure all of this out alone.

How technology ramps up cortisol and causes health problems

**Your phone is making you bigger, more tired, and more anxious —
and it's not even trying to hide it.**

At this point it's hard to do anything without a technological device
involved somewhere. Your phone pulls at your attention constantly —
notifications, texts, email alerts, news alerts, none of them urgent, all of them
activating a low-grade stress response that keeps cortisol quietly elevated
throughout the day. The cumulative effect of this constant interruption is
not trivial. It is a sustained physiological drain that most people have simply
normalized because everyone around them is experiencing the same thing.

The food dimension of this is particularly insidious. Staring at a screen —
phone or television — means being exposed to a continuous stream of food
advertising specifically engineered to trigger cravings and override the part
of your brain that would otherwise make a reasonable decision about dinner.
Door Dash, Uber Eats, and a dozen other apps have made acting on those
cravings friction less. The same device that just showed you an ad for fast
food will now deliver it to your door in thirty minutes, no cooking, no effort,
no nutritional value. And while you're at it, the same phone now offers
prescription medications through apps, with AI increasingly substituting
for the physician conversation that might have asked useful questions —
while the drug advertisements that prompted the visit carefully omit any
mention of the nutritional depletion those prescriptions will cause, further
worsening the cortisol problem they were meant to address.

The calorie picture is equally significant and almost entirely ignored in
public health conversations. Technology hasn't just changed what we eat
— it's changed how much we move while not exercising. Research shows
that non-exercise physical activity can account for up to 2,000 additional
calories burned per day in people who are physically engaged throughout
their lives — cooking, cleaning, running errands, standing instead of
sitting, playing with children and pets, climbing stairs, even singing.[4]
These are not trivial numbers. Daily household activity, done consistently,
often burns more calories than a dedicated gym session. Technology has

systematically replaced most of this activity with sitting, and the metabolic and cortisol consequences are significant, largely unacknowledged, and entirely preventable.

NEAT: Non-Exercise Activity Thermogenesis

Daily calories burned through living vs. screen-based sedentary lifestyle

Active daily living

+2,000

extra cal/day possible

cooking · cleaning · errands
standing · stairs · singing
playing with kids and pets

Screen-based lifestyle

~200

extra cal/day

sitting · scrolling · ordering
delivery apps · screen time
AI robots doing the chores

Why this matters for cortisol

Technology has quietly stolen NEAT — and almost nobody is talking about it.
Daily household activity, done consistently, often burns more calories than a gym session.
NEAT naturally dampens cortisol throughout the day — lower intensity, spread over hours,
without the cortisol spike that high-intensity workouts can produce.

Info graphic 1: NEAT (Non-Exercise Activity Thermogenesis) comparison — bar chart showing active daily living (up to 2,000 extra calories burned) versus sedentary screen-based lifestyle. Activities listed: cooking, cleaning, errands, standing, climbing stairs, playing with children.

Non-exercise activity thermogenesis — the scientific term for all the calories you burn just living your life — is one of the most powerful metabolic tools available to most people, and it costs nothing. It also naturally dampens cortisol in a way that structured exercise sometimes doesn't, because it's lower intensity, spread throughout the day, and doesn't carry the cortisol spike that high-intensity workouts can produce. Technology has quietly stolen this from us, and almost nobody is talking about it.[4]

Then there's what the screens are showing us. The advertising that runs across every platform presents a relentlessly narrow vision of acceptable bodies — the specific shape of a woman, the specific build of a man — that bears no relationship to what healthy human bodies actually look like across age, genetics, and life stage. The psychological toll of this continuous comparison is documented and real. **Body dysmorphia**, disordered eating, and chronic low-level shame about physical appearance are all cortisol drivers in their own right, which means the ads making you feel bad about your body are also making your stress hormones worse. The business model is intact; the health consequences are externalized onto you.

AI adds another layer to this. Beyond the screen-time and advertising problems, AI is now a genuine economic threat for many people — replacing jobs, compressing wages, creating legitimate financial anxiety that has real cortisol consequences. AI-powered housekeeping robots are already commercially available. My advice on that particular development: do your own housecleaning. The physical activity is good for you, the sense of agency over your environment is good for you, and the calories burned are good for you. Outsourcing it to a robot removes all three benefits simultaneously.

The practical prescription

Turn off technology as much as you reasonably can. Turn off the news — it is specifically designed to keep you in a state of low-grade alarm, and the last time it made you feel genuinely better was probably not recently. Reclaim the physical activity that apps and devices have replaced. Cook something. The act of preparing food — the chopping, the stirring, the smell of something on the stove — is itself cortisol-lowering in ways that ordering delivery categorically is not.

Don't fall victim to technology. Your cortisol will thank you.

Poverty drives the damage of cortisol

Everything we've discussed so far gets significantly harder when money is tight.

Food insecurity is a cortisol problem in its most direct form. When you don't know where the next meal is coming from, your stress response isn't a background hum — it's a constant alarm. And the foods most accessible to people in low-income areas tend to be the ones that make cortisol worse: highly processed, calorie-dense, nutrient-poor convenience foods that are cheap, filling, and available when nothing else is. This isn't a failure of willpower or priorities. It's geography, economics, and food system design all converging on the same person at once.

There's also a physiological irony worth understanding here. High-calorie processed foods do temporarily blunt the cortisol response — they provide a brief neurological relief from stress that's completely real, even if short-lived.[5] When that's the only relief available, it makes complete sense that people reach for it. Judging the food choices of people under significant financial stress misses the point entirely.

Food banks fill a genuine gap, though often imperfectly — the quality of available food is frequently limited, which addresses hunger without fully addressing nutrition. Many of my own clients have faced months where food simply ran out before the month did. These are not abstract statistics. They are people managing extraordinary stress with inadequate resources, and the health consequences follow predictably from there.

The research on this is worth taking seriously: food insecurity is meaningfully linked to crime, including violent crime.[5] This isn't a controversial finding — it's a consistent one. Nutritional deprivation affects brain function, impulse regulation, mood stability, and stress tolerance in ways that have downstream consequences for whole communities. When we under invest in food access, we pay for it elsewhere — in emergency rooms, in the justice system, in the compounding costs of preventable chronic disease.

If you're in a position to contribute to food assistance programs, it's one of the highest-leverage things you can do. These programs reduce hospitalizations, support housing stability, and ease pressure on systems that are already stretched. And — not incidentally, given the subject of this book — acts of genuine generosity have a measurable dampening effect on your own cortisol.[5] Helping others, it turns out, is good for your nervous system too.

Your waistline and what it tells you about cortisol

I see it all of the time. My clients struggle to lose weight even when they are meticulous about counting calories. But nothing seems to change the numbers on the scale; they are bloated, and they notice that their waistlines continue to grow no matter what they try. I also hear the stress in their voices, which gives me clues about how to help them: decrease their stress hormones — cortisol — to help them manage their health.

Once my clients are able to address their stress through a functional medicine approach, they almost always notice that their waistlines slim up again. For decades, research has uncovered the vast roles of cortisol in our lives, and one of the major issues that people struggle with is belly fat. Ongoing stress and the cortisol response is related to belly fat.[7]

No prescription medication in the world is equipped to deal with stress-related cortisol. Prescription drugs won't touch the cortisol-gut symptoms either. Finding out the root cause of cortisol and stress in the body can be related to a number of factors, which we will get into next. But it can seem daunting to figure out cortisol levels, as they are rarely checked in conventional medicine.

The other major challenge of stress is that it reduces your ability to absorb nutrients while also making your body burn through nutrients much more quickly than it would if you weren't stressed.[2] Stopping this vicious cycle of nutrient depletion is critical because these nutrients themselves are part of the solution to reducing cortisol and cortisol resistance.

Why conventional medicine misses the mark for cortisol

Turn on the television for twenty minutes and you will almost certainly see an ad for a GLP-1 drug. Happy people on beaches. Effortless weight loss. A life finally under control. The implication is hard to miss: this is the answer, and you've simply been waiting for it.

Here's the more complicated truth. If the underlying driver of your weight gain and health problems is cortisol and nutritional depletion — which, for a significant portion of people struggling with these issues, it is — **GLP-1** drugs won't reach the root cause. They can reduce appetite, sometimes dramatically. But they also deplete nutrients your body is already running short on, which worsens the cortisol problem they were never designed to address in the first place.[2] For many people, the results are genuinely disappointing. Not because the drugs don't work mechanically, but because they're solving for the wrong thing.

The actual root of cortisol-driven weight gain is usually simpler and less photogenic than a beach commercial: nutritional deficiency. Address the deficiencies — through targeted supplementation, whole food nutrition, and stress management — and the weight and cortisol symptoms often begin to resolve without heroic effort. Not always, and not overnight. But more reliably than most people expect, once the underlying depletions are actually corrected.

Magnesium: a place most people need to start

Stress depletes magnesium aggressively and continuously.[2] When cortisol is chronically elevated, your body pulls magnesium directly from bone tissue and excretes it — a process that happens whether or not you're aware of it, and whether or not your doctor has flagged it. This is where the story gets frustrating: magnesium is stored in tissues, not blood, which means standard blood tests look completely normal until depletion is severe. Most people are significantly low in magnesium for years — sometimes decades — before any test reflects it. They ask their doctor, get told their levels are fine, and the deficiency continues entirely unaddressed.

Restoring tissue-level magnesium takes time. Months of consistent supplementation, sometimes longer, depending on how long the depletion has been running. Food sources alone won't close the gap — modern farming has steadily reduced the magnesium content of soil, and two-thirds of foods on grocery shelves have been processed in ways that strip what little remains.[5] Supplementation isn't optional here. It's the only practical way to actually refill what chronic stress has taken.

The payoff is substantial. Magnesium directly dampens cortisol and reduces stress.[2] It improves sleep quality, supports production of serotonin and dopamine, and helps the brain generate **BDNF** — a compound involved in mood, memory, and neurological resilience.[3] With over 300 functions in the body, it is involved in virtually every system that chronic stress disrupts. Low magnesium is independently linked to anxiety, depression, and other mental health conditions.[3] There is even evidence that supplementation reduces aggressive behavior — which, given the current state of things, feels worth mentioning.[8]

Around 300mg daily is a reasonable starting point for most people under significant stress. The form matters, the brand matters, and there are some genuinely unhelpful versions widely available that are worth knowing how to avoid. All of that is covered in Chapter 6 — along with the rest of the nutrients that cortisol depletes and the practical guidance for actually restoring them.

My humbling cortisol-balancing experience with magnesium

A personal account

I'm a dietitian of 26 years, and I like to think of myself as one of the healthcare professionals who keeps on top of my health in all ways. I used to think that I was probably getting enough magnesium if I took a small amount of it in supplements sporadically, especially if I focused on eating magnesium-rich foods. Not so. I didn't realize how much my low magnesium levels were affecting my life in negative ways. Could I have been depleted for many years? I think so. This means that you probably are too, if you aren't supplementing it regularly.

When I honed my magnesium supplement regimen to include 300–500 mg of elemental magnesium with glycine per night, I had pretty dramatic improvements in so many aspects of my health. I'm taking at least three magnesium glycinate capsules per night, or one scoop of magnesium powder at bedtime. After doing so daily and religiously, my stress has dramatically decreased, my sleep has improved, and my mood is much improved. My leg cramps went away, my menstrual cramps decreased, my sugar cravings decreased, and I truly can say I feel so much more relaxed and focused at all points in the day.

What I'm trying to say to you is that you don't know how much better you truly can feel until you try it.

As a dietitian who eats servings of magnesium-rich foods every day — nuts and seeds, leafy greens, dark chocolate, seafood, quinoa, beans, avocados, and dairy — I've learned it still isn't enough. These foods sadly continue to have diminishing amounts of magnesium as modern farming practices have caused soil levels to be increasingly low in magnesium. The lesson: if someone who eats as well as I do is still significantly depleted, the rest of the stressed, busy, processed-food-eating population almost certainly is too.

The magnesium depletion-stress cycle

Graphic 2: Magnesium depletion cycle — circular diagram showing: Chronic stress → cortisol spike → magnesium pulled from bones and excreted → tissue depletion → blood test reads "normal" → deficiency goes unaddressed → cortisol worsens. Exit point: magnesium glycinate supplementation 300–500mg at bedtime.

References

1 Perry BD, et al. The cost of child maltreatment. *Child Welfare.* 1997. https://pubmed.ncbi.nlm.nih.gov/10798840/

2 Pickering G, et al. Magnesium status and stress: The vicious circle concept revisited. *Nutrients.* 2020. https://www.mdpi.com/2072-6643/12/12/3672

3 Botturi A, et al. The role and effect of magnesium in mental disorders. *Nutrients.* 2020. https://www.frontiersin.org/journals/psychiatry/articles/

10.3389/fpsyt.2023.1176061/full

4 von Loeffelholz C, Birkenfeld AL. Non-exercise activity thermogenesis. In: *Endotext*. MDText.com; 2022. https://www.ncbi.nlm.nih.gov/books/NBK279077/

5 Food insecurity and crime. *BMC Public Health*. 2021. https://pubmed.ncbi.nlm.nih.gov/34676506/

6 Dallman MF, et al. Chronic stress, obesity, and comfort food. *Proc Natl Acad Sci USA*. 2003. https://pubmed.ncbi.nlm.nih.gov/11020091/

7 Epel ES, et al. Stress and body shape: cortisol secretion and central fat. *Psychosom Med*. 2000. https://pubmed.ncbi.nlm.nih.gov/27345309/

8 Semaglutide and nutritional deficiency. *J Clin Endocrinol Metab*. 2025. https://www.sciencedirect.com/science/article/pii/S2667368125000

3

Chapter 3

SUPPORTIVE WAYS TO REDUCE STRESS AND CORTISOL FROM TRAUMA

As a dietitian and nutritionist, I can talk about food and nutrients all day and how they help reduce stress. This, in my experience, can't be overlooked. But it can't be a standalone approach for people who have experienced a lot of life stress and trauma. Experts in the field of trauma, such as Bessel van der Kolk, author of *The Body Keeps the Score*, are great resources for understanding the best options for managing PTSD. In this chapter, you will learn some effective strategies to help you balance your life and, by doing so, balance your cortisol levels. These strategies can include clinical **hypnotherapy**, acupuncture, **EMDR**, social support, meditation, and more.

Hypnotherapy: a misunderstood but highly effective way to reduce cortisol

Using hypnotherapy with a highly skilled clinical hypnotherapist is often my go-to strategy to help my clients heal from their stress and trauma in the quickest way. I've had personal and profound improvements in my own health that have lasted for 10 years, and counting, from a few sessions of hypnotherapy from a wonderful hypnotherapist, Clark Patton. These sessions are simply transformative in the best ways because they help the subconscious brain overcome deep wounds quickly.[1,2,3]

All the talk therapy in the world can't compare to these powerful tools we can harness when we learn that our relaxed state is the preferred state that our brain wants to be in. But when talk therapy is combined with hypnotherapy, the combination is exceptionally powerful for healing traumas and even helping people with complex PTSD, according to the *American Journal of Hypnotherapy*.[1] In the 1990s, the *Journal of Clinical Psychiatry* described the many benefits of hypnotherapy for helping people with stress and trauma.[3] Hypnotherapy isn't often recommended by the conventional medical model, but it should be.

Why I recommend hypnotherapy first

Of all the tools in this chapter, hypnotherapy is the one I reach for most consistently with clients dealing with deep-rooted stress and trauma. The results are faster, more durable, and more complete than any other single intervention I've used. A few sessions with a skilled practitioner can accomplish what years of talk therapy sometimes cannot — because hypnotherapy bypasses the analytical mind entirely and works directly with the subconscious patterns that are driving the cortisol response.

To find a skilled clinical hypnotherapist, look for someone with CHt (Certified Hypnotherapist) credentials and specific experience with stress and trauma. Ask about their approach before booking.

Hypnosis and the question of control

The following reflection is contributed by Clark Patton, CHt. I'll let Clark explain what actually happens in that hypnotherapy session — because frankly, he does it better than I can.

There is a lens we could look at the mind and body through: the idea of control. Many clients come to me because they are encountering an absence of control, either mentally or physically. Really, we can't look at the two as separate. Our physical body affects our mind, and each thought we have sends a cascade of chemical signals that directly affect our body. To look at one without the other would be a mistake.

The loss of control in the physical sense is often tied to an overactive nervous system. The nervous system has two main modes that it works in: the **sympathetic** and the **parasympathetic nervous system**. The autonomic nervous system is commonly referred to as the "fight or flight" mode. This mode is meant to be used sparingly, during times of stress, danger, or excitement. When it's engaged, the heart rate and blood pressure go up, breathing becomes more shallow, and blood often moves away from the vital organs to the muscles and extremities. Things like digestion and reproduction slow down, because they are not vital during survival mode. Unfortunately, our society mainly encourages this mode, and we see an expanding epidemic of stress and anxiety. All sorts of ailments — both physical and mental — can stem from here, ranging from digestive issues to fatigue, persistent worry, panic attacks, brain fog, autoimmune flare-ups, muscle tension, weight issues, and much more. Surprisingly, the answer for many clients I work with is actually to "do less" to achieve the balance their body needs.

As soon as we tap into a more relaxed flow state, the overall level of energy our body requires goes down, and yet there are huge improvements in performance. We utilize more of the parasympathetic nervous system, which brings a natural balance and allows the body to do what it knows how to do. The question we must ask ourselves is: "If I'm not able to let go of control when I want to or need to... am I really in control?" It is letting go at the right time that really benefits us. Tapping into a part of ourselves that uses less energy for better results is ideal. In fact, this is what our bodies are designed to do! Our hunter-gatherer predecessors did not get us here by squandering calories, but by using the least amount of effort for the best results.

Once clients tap into this natural part of themselves, they begin to see tremendous results, not only in the main areas that are problematic, but also the effects ripple into other aspects of their life. A person who is depressed — often resulting from longstanding anxiety — not only escapes sadness but may also start to feel a surge of motivation as their energies are freed up. Or perhaps they start to find enjoyment in daily life again. They begin to send themselves on an upward spiral, gaining momentum… how far a person takes it is up to them, and their trajectory is within their control.

Hypnotherapy is a unique tool for accessing these problems. It directly affects the nervous system in a very beneficial way, allowing people to tap into their parasympathetic nervous system. The process involves collapsing and resolving unhealthy patterns from the past, while also building the future responses we want to have. In my opinion, hypnotherapy encompasses many other healing modalities: EMDR, biofeedback, **Neuro Linguistic Programming**, meditation and mindfulness, somatic therapy, and cognitive behavioral therapy (to name a few). The common thread in all these methods is that they seek to bypass the analytical, logical mind. However, unlike some of these other methods, hypnosis seeks to put the tools in the hands of the client so they can continue to affect their life without needing anyone else to do it. So many of the ailments people struggle with have nothing to do with logic. In a meditative (hypnotic) state, a person interacts with the part of themselves that does not operate analytically, but rather through association.

As far as I can tell, people rarely become the way they are by accident. An experienced practitioner has the experience and understanding of patterns to recognize this. Our experiences, associations, and underlying beliefs form the automatic responses we experience. The truth is, as long as we are capable of learning new skills, things can be different for us. As a hypnotherapist, I seek to expand people's options and find the best avenue to pursue.

How we learn a new skill/response:

1. We are unaware that we are even experiencing a problem.
2. We become aware that there is a problem, but we don't know how to fix it.
3. We learn why the problem is happening and what is needed to resolve it.
4. We use this solution until it is a part of us — automatic.

When a person uses hypnosis to address something new they want in their life, it is this same process… just sped up. What we want is for the automatic mind/body to no longer be our opponent, but instead something that aligns and effectively works with us. It is not uncommon for some clients I work with to successfully go through all these stages in an hour and a half, creating long-lasting shifts in their life. Other times, it requires further reinforcement as people need to build their experiences and successes for a new pattern to be fully established. The result is transformation. The goal is not to change the person, but to help them become more themselves than ever before.

Ultimately, we control the trajectory of our life, despite external challenges that we navigate. Our mind can improve, our body can improve… continuously. In fact, we need them to! What we once imagined was impossible can become something automatic — a part of us. Each individual is so wildly unique that I find healing and progress rarely looks the same for any two people. We have the control and the choice to embrace this path; hypnosis is a tool along the way. In this process we don't give up control, but rather we reclaim it.

Sympathetic vs. parasympathetic nervous system

Sympathetic Fight or flight — cortisol activated	Parasympathetic Rest and digest — cortisol normalized
↑ Heart rate and blood pressure	↓ Calm heart rate and pressure
↑ Shallow, rapid breathing	↓ Deep, slow breathing
↓ Digestion slows or stops	↑ Digestion active and efficient
↑ Cortisol and adrenaline spike	↓ Cortisol at healthy baseline
↓ Reproduction and immunity	↑ Healing and immune function
Modern life keeps us here chronically	**Hypnotherapy activates this state**

The goal of every intervention in this chapter is to shift left → right

Diagram 1: Sympathetic vs. parasympathetic nervous system comparison — two-column visual showing fight-or-flight responses (elevated heart rate, shallow breathing, digestion slowed, cortisol spiked) versus rest-and-digest responses (calm heart rate, deep breathing, digestion active, cortisol normalized). Hypnotherapy shown as pathway to parasympathetic activation.

Acupuncture for trauma and cortisol

Most people who have tried **acupuncture** will tell you that it is a helpful and balancing experience. It feels quite relaxing and is a technique used for thousands of years to help heal many imbalances in the body. As part of **Traditional Chinese Medicine**, acupuncture is not easy to quantify because it helps balance whole-body systems and is not designed to target cortisol levels per se. Nonetheless, some studies show that acupuncture helps reduce cortisol levels, as is the case in people recovering from knee surgery and in people with high levels of stress.[4,5] Acupuncture also reduces PTSD symptoms according to some research.[6]

My observations over the years are that acupuncture, in general, is a highly effective way to help deal with pain and suffering of many kinds. It can help people avoid dangerous pain medications and anxiety medications. Clearly, some acupuncturists are more highly skilled than others, so do your homework to find a good one in your area. But I don't think it can be a standalone remedy for healing cortisol issues: people should address core deficiencies in the body, imbalances in the body, and build supportive social lives.

Stress and EMDR

EMDR, or Eye Movement Desensitization and Reprocessing, can be useful for people with high levels of stress. It's easy to study, so that is why you will find a lot of mental health therapists use it. But I personally find that hypnotherapy has a much stronger and quicker benefit for people with long-term stress and anxiety. Research is somewhat disappointing in terms of the effects of EMDR on cortisol. One study found that EMDR does not reduce cortisol levels;[7] however, another study found that "treatment responders" had a reduction in cortisol after EMDR use,[8] so it is likely to help some people more than others.

Don't get me wrong — EMDR can be highly useful and I use it myself. I suggest learning about EMDR yourself. Here is a quick EMDR exercise on YouTube worth trying: https://www.youtube.com/watch?v=CdFQwL08Yd w&t=12s

Supportive friends

An important tool for managing stress and trauma is connecting with supportive friends and family, working with collaborative people, and social support. Anything that helps you live in the present will help get you on the path to recovery, and this is why supportive friends and family are critical. In *The Body Keeps the Score* (van der Kolk, 2015), the importance of healthy social connections is emphasized many times. While these connections can be somewhat challenging to find when you are stressed, they are a cornerstone of managing cortisol that can't be overlooked. I suggest that you read or listen to this book to see how powerful these connections are.

Cortisol thrives in isolation. Connection is its antidote.

Meditation and gentle exercise

Meditation and mind-body therapies like yoga, dance, and gentle physical activity are essential for managing day-to-day issues with stress and cortisol. An important fact that you should know is that when you are meditating, you are in a state of hypnosis. Tools that can help you meditate include slow breathing techniques, body scan meditations, and more. You can find useful tools for free on YouTube as well. But you should be aware that strenuous exercise drives up your body's cortisol levels, at least temporarily. This could be in part because strenuous exercise depletes the body of nutrients.[11]

Free resources to help you meditate

I personally love using body scan meditation and the meditation videos on YouTube. I suggest checking out the work by Michael Seeley. I also recommend reading the book *Breath: The New Science of a Lost Art* by James Nestor. Simple but powerful breathing techniques described in this book can help your body enter a zen state and lower your cortisol naturally.

Gentle exercises like yoga and dance help us feel grounded in our bodies. A lot of the issues with chronic stress is that we lose the ability to stay grounded. But some exercises are better for reducing cortisol than others. Yoga results in a stronger improvement in mood and a stronger reduction in anxiety than walking.[9] Dance also is effective at reducing anxiety, and it is my personal favorite form of exercise because of the integration of movement and music.[10]

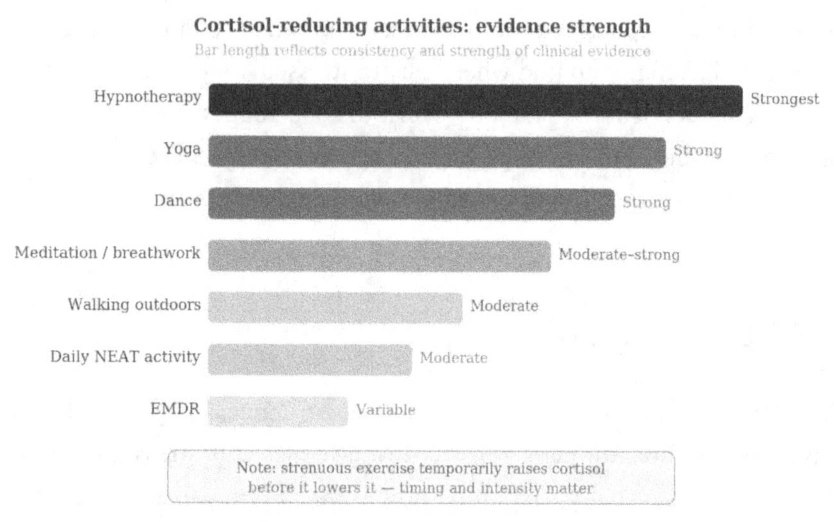

Comparison chart: Cortisol-reducing activities ranked by evidence strength — horizontal bar chart showing Hypnotherapy (strongest evidence), Yoga, Dance, Meditation/breath work, Walking, Gentle housework/NEAT, EMDR (variable). Note: strenuous exercise temporarily raises cortisol before lowering it.

Don't just get by — get restorative sleep for cortisol balance

I have a complicated relationship with sleep.

Not in the way that sounds dramatic — I function, I've always functioned —

but for most of my childhood and well into adulthood, sleep was something that happened to other people while I lay in the dark cataloging everything I'd said wrong, or wrongs done to me, that day. The mental replays, the low-grade guilt, the thoughts that seemed perfectly reasonable at 2am and completely absurd by morning. Classic subconscious overtime. As I've since learned, it was also directly connected to what I was eating — childhood food preferences that were keeping my cortisol unbalanced in ways I wouldn't understand for years.

I'm telling you this because I want you to know that the sleep advice in this section isn't theoretical. It's hard-won.

The single most effective thing I've found for sleep — for myself and for my clients — isn't a supplement or a sleep tracker or a magnesium-infused pillow mist. It's addressing what's running underneath. The subconscious patterns, the unresolved stress, the mind that won't stop composing emails at midnight. A skilled clinical hypnotherapist is the fastest route I know to getting that under control, as I discussed in the previous section. If that feels like a big step right now, a good body scan meditation on YouTube costs nothing and works better than most people expect. Start there.

Nutrients come next — and they matter more than most people realize for sleep specifically. Magnesium is the cornerstone: it regulates the neurotransmitters that wind the nervous system down at night, and most stressed people are significantly depleted in it. Herbs fill in the gaps beautifully. Chapters 6 and 7 cover both in detail, but the short version is that fixing your nutrient status at night changes the quality of sleep in ways that feel almost immediate once you experience it.

The caffeine conversation nobody wants to have

If you are regularly tired, regularly stressed, and regularly reaching for coffee to close the gap, the coffee may be part of why the gap keeps growing. Caffeine disrupts **REM sleep** — the deep, restorative phase that your brain uses to process emotion, consolidate memory, and regulate stress hormones — even when you don't feel like it's affecting your sleep at all.[12] You fall asleep fine. You stay asleep. But the quality is compromised in ways that accumulate quietly, leaving you more tired and more cortisol-reactive the next day, which then sends you back to the coffee, which then disrupts the next night's sleep.

It's a tidy little cycle. And it's worth breaking.

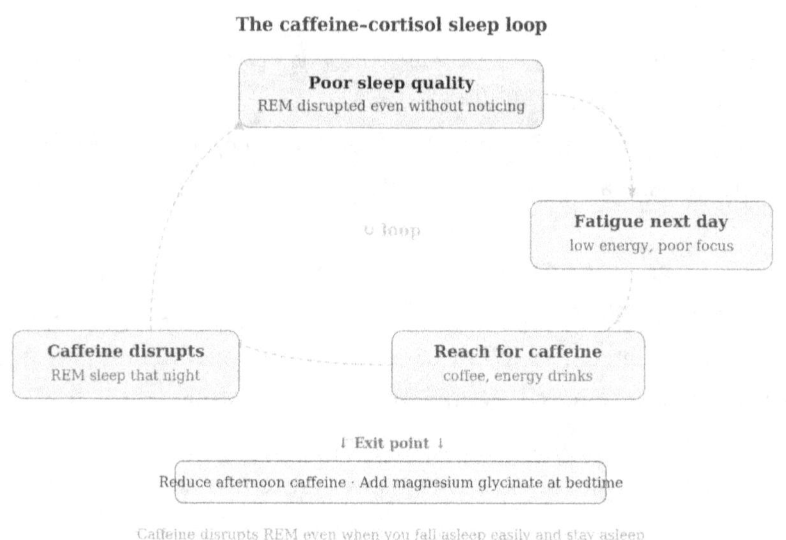

Diagram: The caffeine-cortisol sleep loop — circular: Poor sleep quality → fatigue next day → reach for caffeine → caffeine disrupts REM → poor sleep quality. Exit point shown: reduce afternoon/evening caffeine, add magnesium glycinate at bedtime.

Antidepressant prescriptions: a double-edged sword for cortisol and weight?

Let's have an honest conversation about antidepressants — one that doesn't end with either "they're a lifesaver" or "they're poison," because the truth, as usual, is more interesting than either extreme.

Antidepressants and mood stabilizers genuinely help a lot of people. That's real and worth saying clearly. But there's a significant footnote that almost nobody mentions at the prescribing appointment: many of these medications quietly deplete the nutrients your body needs to regulate mood in the first place.[17] **SSRIs**, for example, interfere with the body's ability to produce niacin — vitamin B3 — a nutrient directly involved in stress metabolism. Other B vitamins, including folate and B12, are depleted enough by some medications that researchers have found supplementing them actually improves how well the antidepressants work.[17] Which raises an obvious question: how many people are on sub optimal doses of medication, or cycling through different prescriptions, when part of the problem is a nutrient deficiency the medication itself created?

This is not an argument against medication. It's an argument for knowing what your medication is doing to your nutritional status, and compensating accordingly.

Vitamin D and mood: the overlooked connection

Speaking of nutrients and mood — vitamin D deserves its own moment here. It's not glamorous. It doesn't have a pharmaceutical marketing budget. But a review of 25 clinical trials found that vitamin D supplementation meaningfully reduces negative emotions, particularly in people with low blood levels — which, given that most people are deficient, is most people.[13] Part of the mechanism is straightforward: vitamin D helps the body produce serotonin, the same neurotransmitter that SSRIs are designed to preserve.[14] It also directly influences cortisol production.[14] The side effect profile in moderate doses is essentially nothing. It costs almost nothing. And yet it remains almost completely absent from the standard depression conversation.

The SSRI weight gain problem

Now for the part about SSRIs that really should be mentioned upfront — and almost never is.

Roughly half of people who take SSRIs gain weight.[15] Half. This isn't a rare side effect buried in the fine print — it's a coin flip. The mechanism isn't fully understood, but emerging research suggests SSRIs may impair **mitochondrial** function — the cellular machinery responsible for burning calories.[16] Whether that damage is reversible with long-term use remains genuinely unknown.[16] And weight gain, for many people, is itself a significant source of stress, low self-esteem, and worsening mood — which rather complicates the picture of a medication prescribed to improve those exact things.

None of this means medication is wrong for you. For some people it's absolutely the right tool, and removing it without guidance would be both dangerous and unnecessary. But "medication is appropriate for many people" and "medication is the only option worth discussing" are two very different statements, and conventional medicine has a tendency to treat them as the same.

Evidence-based natural alternatives

There are evidence-based alternatives worth knowing about. Saffron — not the spice you forgot you bought two years ago, but supplemental saffron at affordable and therapeutic doses — has been shown across multiple clinical trials to reduce depression symptoms comparably to SSRIs, without the weight gain or the mitochondrial question marks.[17] Turmeric and other anti-inflammatory compounds address what may be the most underappreciated driver of depression: systemic inflammation. When you reduce inflammation, you frequently get a brain that functions better — not because you've masked a symptom, but because you've addressed a cause.

Saffron: the mood spice with clinical credentials

Six clinical trials have confirmed saffron's effectiveness for anxiety and depression — comparable results to SSRIs, without the weight gain, sexual dysfunction, or suicidal ideation that appear in the SSRI side effect list.[17] SSRIs have existed for about 40 years. Saffron has been used for several thousand. The evidence base for "we don't know enough about herbs" is getting harder to defend with a straight face.

More on saffron at thehealthyrd.com/saffrons-fascinating-benefits

When to seek help

It is always important to get help for stress and cortisol if either is interfering with your daily life. If you feel overwhelmed and your symptoms of cortisol are unrelenting, you should seek advice from your healthcare team. This team can include many types of therapists, including talk therapy, acupuncture, hypnotherapy, and holistic providers of many kinds.

Chapter 3 summary: your cortisol-reducing toolkit

- **Hypnotherapy** — fastest and most durable results for deep trauma and chronic stress; seek a CHt-credentialed practitioner
- **Acupuncture** — cortisol-lowering and PTSD-reducing; works best alongside nutritional support
- **EMDR** — useful for some; results vary; can be combined with hypnotherapy for stronger effect
- **Social connection** — non-negotiable; cortisol thrives in isolation
- **Yoga and dance** — stronger cortisol reduction than walking; dance is particularly effective for trauma integration
- **Sleep hygiene** — address subconscious patterns first, then nutrients, then caffeine

- **Nutritional support for antidepressant users** — supplement B vitamins, vitamin D, and consider saffron as a natural adjunct

References

1 Alladin A. Hypnotherapy for complex PTSD. *Am J Clin Hypn.* 2025. https://pubmed.ncbi.nlm.nih.gov/39908116/

2 Alladin A, Alibhai A. Cognitive hypnotherapy for depression. *Int J Clin Exp Hypn.* 2007. https://pubmed.ncbi.nlm.nih.gov/33118880/

3 Spiegel D. Hypnosis and traumatic dissociation. *J Trauma Dissociation.* 1991. https://pubmed.ncbi.nlm.nih.gov/2211565/

4 Meng X, et al. Acupuncture and cortisol in knee surgery recovery. *Front Endocrinol.* 2023. https://pubmed.ncbi.nlm.nih.gov/37920858/

5 Eshkevari L, et al. Acupuncture and HPA axis components. *J Endocrinol.* 2020. https://pmc.ncbi.nlm.nih.gov/articles/PMC7377446/

6 Engel CC, et al. Acupuncture for PTSD. *Med Care.* 2024. https://pubmed.ncbi.nlm.nih.gov/38381417/

7 Sack M, et al. EMDR and cortisol. *Psychother Psychosom.* 2008. https://pubmed.ncbi.nlm.nih.gov/29171317/

8 Schubert SJ, et al. Cortisol outcomes after EMDR. *Eur J Psychotraumatol.* 2016. https://pmc.ncbi.nlm.nih.gov/articles/PMC2880549/

9 Streeter CC, et al. Yoga versus walking and anxiety. *J Altern Complement Med.* 2010. https://pmc.ncbi.nlm.nih.gov/articles/PMC3111147/

10 Eyigor S, et al. Dance and anxiety reduction. *Int J Nurs Stud.* 1984. https://pubmed.ncbi.nlm.nih.gov/6473025/

11 Heffernan SM, et al. Strenuous exercise and mineral depletion. *Biol Trace Elem Res.* 2009. https://link.springer.com/article/10.1007/s12011-008-8217-5

12 Weibel J, et al. Caffeine and REM sleep. *Nutrients.* 2021. https://pmc.ncbi.nlm.nih.gov/articles/PMC8276335/

13 Shaffer JA, et al. Vitamin D and depression. *Nutrients.* 2025. https://pmc.ncbi.nlm.nih.gov/articles/PMC11872774/

14 Vitamin D and cortisol production. *Clin Nutr Res.* 2025. https://www.sciencedirect.com/science/article/pii/S2666396125000615

15 Serretti A, Mandelli L. Antidepressants and body weight. *J Clin Psychiatry.* 2010. https://www.sciencedirect.com/science/article/abs/pii/S0163834314002837

16 Tobe EH. Mitochondrial dysfunction and depression. *Neuropsychiatr Dis Treat.* 2013. https://pubmed.ncbi.nlm.nih.gov/21120605/

17 Lopresti AL, et al. Saffron and antidepressant effects. *J Affect Disord.* 2019. https://pubmed.ncbi.nlm.nih.gov/31423805/

4

Chapter 4

WHICH CAME FIRST — THE INFLAMMATION OR THE HIGH CORTISOL?

Here's cortisol's most maddening trick:

The same hormone your body releases to fight inflammation will, if it stays elevated long enough, cause more inflammation. Not less. More.

Take a moment with that one.

It explains why chronically stressed people feel simultaneously wired and exhausted, inflamed and depleted — the alarm system meant to help is now part of the problem. It also explains why prednisone, the synthetic cortisol doctors prescribe for inflammatory conditions, works beautifully in the short term and creates a fairly spectacular mess over time. The cortisol goes up, the inflammation eventually goes up with it, the body stops responding to cortisol properly, and everyone wonders why nothing is getting better.

KEY INSIGHT

The cortisol-inflammation paradox: Cortisol is released to suppress inflammation. But when cortisol stays chronically elevated, it eventually causes more inflammation — not less. This is one of the most important and most overlooked facts in stress medicine.

The cortisol-inflammation loop

An interesting phenomenon happens when you have elevated cortisol levels, from prescriptions or otherwise: over the long term, **inflammation** increases. This is a bit of a conundrum, but is real nonetheless. And another intriguing problem exists. When you have inflammation in your body from an unhealthy diet, this inflammation causes the release of cortisol in an effort to balance out the inflammation. Elevated cortisol due to inflammation creates **cortisol resistance**, so your body's cortisol essentially stops functioning effectively.

The solution to balancing cortisol can be rather simple: dampen inflammation by healing your gut and eating **anti-inflammatory** foods and herbs. However, our society doesn't exactly promote anti-inflammatory foods and herbs. In the 1920s, the Flexner Report helped pharmaceutical interests quietly reorganize medicine around patentable treatments and away from everything that grew in the ground.[3] If that sounds conspiratorial, read the report. It's not subtle.

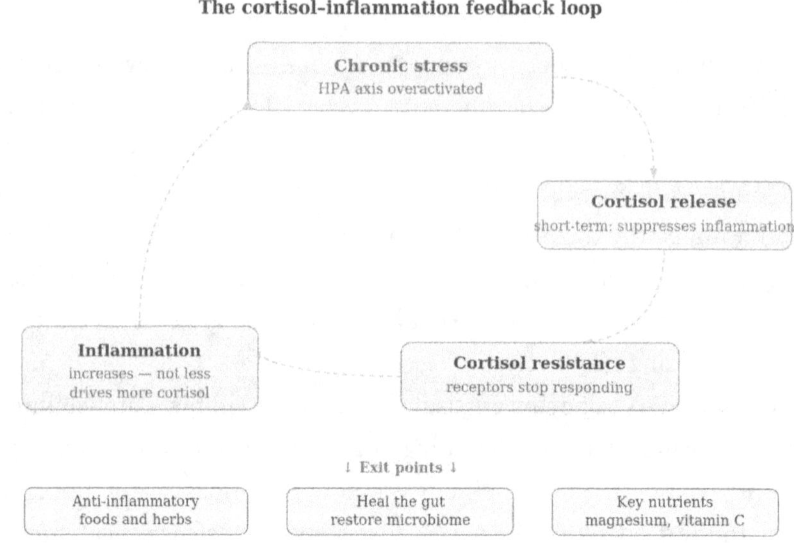

Diagram 1: The cortisol-inflammation feedback loop — circular diagram: Chronic stress → cortisol release → short-term inflammation suppression → prolonged cortisol elevation → cortisol resistance → inflammation increases → more cortisol released → loop continues. Exit points shown: anti-inflammatory foods, gut healing, herbs.

Herbal options: more powerful than most people expect

The herbal options in particular are more powerful than most people expect. Lavender — yes, the one in candles — is also an edible herb with documented anti-inflammatory properties that reduces cortisol release by 70% in clinical research.[2] Seventy percent. Tulsi, saffron, and chamomile work through similar pathways. Six clinical trials have confirmed saffron's effectiveness for anxiety and depression specifically — comparable results to SSRIs, without the weight gain, sexual dysfunction, or suicidal ideation that show up in the SSRI side effect list.[3] SSRIs have existed for about 40 years. Saffron has been used for several thousand. The evidence base for "we don't know enough about herbs" is getting harder to defend with a straight face.

Lavender: the 70% cortisol reduction nobody talks about

In a study of 90 patients preparing for heart surgery — a population under about as much acute stress as it's possible to be under — inhaling lavender essential oil reduced cortisol levels by 70% compared to the control group.[2] That's not a subtle effect. That's a dramatic, measurable reduction in the primary stress hormone from aromatherapy alone.

And part of the reason that herbs like saffron, lavender, and tulsi work to help mood is that they naturally help dampen inflammation in the body while restoring balance and even helping with memory — without the side effect profiles that pharmaceutical alternatives carry.

Healing the gut: the gatekeeper of inflammation

Healing the gut is paramount to reducing inflammation. This is because the gut is the gatekeeper for our body from the outside world and the gatekeeper of inflammation. By eating nutritious foods the way nature intended them to be, our bodies are able to calm down the inflammatory response in a holistic way. The gut is responsible for almost all of our body's inflammatory response because it is also responsible for most of our immune system. This is why eliminating gut triggers and eating healing foods is so critical to your whole body. Your gut triggers can be different from mine, but on the whole, the most common food triggers for gut issues are gluten, soy, legumes, dairy, corn, shellfish, and processed foods. But when you heal the gut, your body may be able to tolerate small amounts of your specific trigger foods.

There can be a lot to healing the gut, as I discuss in my book *Gut Fix*. But the core principle is consistent: reduce the inflammatory triggers, restore beneficial bacteria, heal the gut lining, and cortisol management becomes dramatically more achievable.

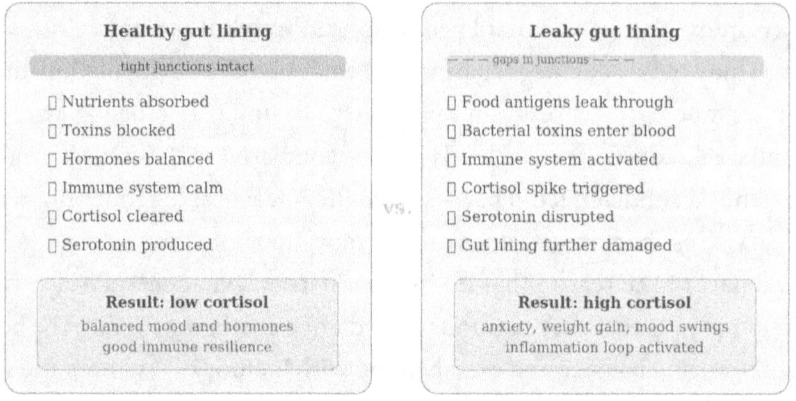

Diagram 2: The gut as inflammation gatekeeper — cross-section showing intact gut lining (healthy: nutrients absorbed, toxins blocked, hormones balanced) versus leaky gut lining (inflamed: food antigens leak through, immune activation, cortisol spike). Common food triggers listed alongside: gluten, dairy, soy, corn, legumes, shellfish, processed foods.

Agricultural chemicals: the inflammation driver nobody warned you about

You should know that chemicals sprayed on foods cause inflammation. The situation continues to get worse. **Glyphosate** — the active ingredient in Roundup, sprayed on most conventionally grown wheat, corn, soy, oats, and legumes — has been the subject of over 100,000 legal claims and more than $11 billion in settlements against Monsanto.[5,6] The company also funded research concluding their own product was safe, which is the kind of conflict of interest that would be funny if the health consequences weren't so serious.[5] Their response to mounting legal pressure has been to shift toward **glufosinate** — a different chemical, similar concerns, and a fresh 30-year window before the lawsuits catch up.[4]

There is no meaningful oversight of these chemical companies. Yet it is still legal on the market — a telling sign of corruption that goes deep.

The Monsanto timeline worth knowing

- **Glyphosate (Roundup)** — sprayed on most conventionally grown grains and legumes; subject to over 100,000 health-related legal claims; $11+ billion in settlements
- **Fake safety studies** — Monsanto paid scientists to produce research declaring glyphosate "safe," subsequently exposed
- **Glufosinate** — the replacement chemical now being applied as glyphosate litigation grows; health research is sparse, concerns are significant
- **Organic foods** — measurably reduce inflammatory chemical burden within 5 days of switching

You shouldn't stress over this for obvious reasons — stress makes everything worse. But consider that the cost gap between organic and conventional foods has narrowed considerably. It's worth checking in your own grocery store if you last looked a while ago.

Buying organic: a meaningful and practical step

Please buy organic foods if you can to help your cortisol levels and to reduce inflammation in your body. You shouldn't stress over this for obvious reasons — stress makes everything worse. But consider the fact that conventionally grown foods have dramatically increased in cost while organic foods haven't kept pace, narrowing the gap in costs. A recent study showed that if you choose organic foods, it can reduce the chemical inflammatory burden in your body in as little as 5 days.[7]

Five days is not a long time to wait for a meaningful change. This isn't about perfection — it's about direction. Every shift toward organic, whole, unprocessed food reduces the inflammatory burden that is driving your cortisol response.

Buy the organic carrots, take a breath, and keep going.

Antioxidants stop the fire of inflammation

There is a lot of proof that inflammation drives cortisol and stress, so are **anti-inflammatory** foods the answer? **Antioxidants** help to improve our body's response to cortisol.[8] The same goes for anti-inflammatory compounds and the insulin response, and likely all other hormones like thyroid hormone and sex hormones.[9] If you have a lot of inflammation from your diet, you likely aren't receiving any of your hormone messages properly. Antioxidant foods and nutrients help to enhance this hormone messaging in the body. But if you've been on a cortisol roller coaster for a long time, your body's reserves for antioxidants and nutrients are depleted.[10,11] Similarly, inflammatory foods can be the root cause of your stress and cortisol. To recover, you will want to take a close look at your diet, supplement regimen, and lifestyle. I will help you make these choices as we go through this book.

Anti-inflammatory foods and cortisol

Choose these to break the inflammation-cortisol loop

Fatty fish

Omega-3 fatty acids directly reduce baseline cortisol levels

salmon · sardines · mackerel cod · trout

Colorful vegetables

Antioxidants reduce oxidative stress and restore hormone sensitivity

beets · peppers · sweet potato leafy greens · broccoli

Fermented foods

Probiotics balance the gut-cortisol loop and restore microbiome

kefir · sauerkraut · kimchi yogurt · miso

Herbs and spices

GABA enhancement, direct cortisol reduction through multiple pathways

rosemary · turmeric · ginger lavender · sage · chamomile

Organic whole grains

Steady glucose prevents cortisol spikes from blood sugar crashes

wild rice · quinoa · oats sourdough · organic rye

Avoid these

Drive inflammation and worsen cortisol loop

seed oils · processed foods glyphosate-sprayed grains refined sugar

Switch to organic foods: reduces chemical inflammatory burden within 5 days
Antioxidant-rich eating restores hormone sensitivity across all hormones

Info graphic: Anti-inflammatory food categories and their cortisol-balancing effects — showing fatty fish (omega-3s, reduce baseline cortisol), colorful vegetables (antioxidants, reduce oxidative stress), fermented foods (probiotics, balance gut-cortisol loop), herbs and spices (GABA enhancement, direct cortisol reduction), organic whole grains (steady glucose, prevent cortisol spikes). Contrasted against: seed oils, processed foods, glyphosate-sprayed grains.

Chapter 4 summary

Key takeaways

- **The cortisol-inflammation paradox is real.** Cortisol suppresses inflammation short-term but causes more inflammation long-term. This is why chronically stressed people feel simultaneously wired and sick.

- **The gut is ground zero.** Most inflammation originates in the gut. Healing the gut is the single most impactful step you can take to break the cortisol-inflammation cycle.
- **Agricultural chemicals are a hidden driver.** Glyphosate disrupts GABA, damages gut lining, and drives inflammation. Switching to organic food measurably reduces chemical inflammatory burden within 5 days.
- **Herbs work — and the evidence is solid.** Lavender (70% cortisol reduction), saffron (comparable to SSRIs), tulsi, and chamomile all dampen inflammation and cortisol through multiple overlapping pathways.
- **Antioxidant-rich foods restore hormone sensitivity.** Chronic inflammation impairs the body's ability to receive hormone signals properly. Anti-inflammatory eating restores this sensitivity across all hormones, not just cortisol.

In the next chapters, I devote a lot of time helping you reduce cortisol by fixing what is on your plate — and what is in your supplement cabinet.

References

1 Cain DW, Cidlowski JA. Immune regulation by glucocorticoids. *Nat Rev Immunol.* 2017. https://pmc.ncbi.nlm.nih.gov/articles/PMC3178858/

2 Vakili S, et al. Lavender aromatherapy reduces cortisol by 70%. *Complement Ther Med.* 2015. https://pubmed.ncbi.nlm.nih.gov/27563324/

3 SSRI long-term side effects. *Prim Care Companion CNS Disord.* 2003. https://pmc.ncbi.nlm.nih.gov/articles/PMC181155/

4 Cooper A, et al. Glufosinate and health risks. *Environ Health Perspect.* 2020. https://pubmed.ncbi.nlm.nih.gov/32578317/

5 Portier CJ, et al. Industry influence and glyphosate safety studies. *Environ Health.* 2022. https://pmc.ncbi.nlm.nih.gov/articles/PMC9229215/

6 Monsanto Roundup lawsuit updates. https://www.sokolovelaw.com/product-liability/monsanto-roundup/lawsuit-updates/

7 Katz DL, et al. Organic diet and reduction of chemical exposure. *J Hum Environ*. 2012. https://pubmed.ncbi.nlm.nih.gov/32797996/

8 Kim JH, et al. Antioxidants and cortisol response. *Nutrients*. 2016. https://pmc.ncbi.nlm.nih.gov/articles/PMC4783970/

9 Dembek M, et al. Anti-inflammatory antioxidants and insulin resistance. *Front Endocrinol*. 2014. https://pmc.ncbi.nlm.nih.gov/articles/PMC3978663/

10 Lucassen PJ, et al. Glucocorticoids and oxidative stress. *Int J Neuropsychopharmacol*. 2008. https://academic.oup.com/ijnp/article/11/6/851/671366

11 Antioxidants and HPA axis function. *Nutrients*. 2016. https://pmc.ncbi.nlm.nih.gov/articles/PMC3325609/

5

Chapter 5

BUILDING CORTISOL-BUSTING MEALS

Nutrition plays a critical role in maintaining our **gut health**, which is directly tied to hormone production and release, including cortisol.[1] A nutrient-rich diet fosters a healthy gut microbiome and healthy cortisol levels, influencing both physical health and mental well-being. This is a two-way street. The better your physical health is, the better your mental health is, and the more resilient you can be from life stressors. Nutrients and diet factors also directly support mental and physical well-being by increasing hormone sensitivity, hormone balance, and thus support balanced cortisol levels. In this chapter, learn how to reduce cortisol levels by supporting your body with healthy meals and making your meals a stress-free zone.

The basics of cortisol-friendly meal planning

Gut bacteria can make or break your mental health, as we discussed previously. If you eat a diverse, nutrient-rich diet, you can promote a more varied and healthy gut bacterial community. This in turn can support your immune function, dampen inflammation, improve mental health, and overall well-being. And the best part about all of this is that healthy gut bacteria regulate your fight-or-flight hormone — cortisol.[1] Fermented foods, fiber-rich fruits and vegetables, healthy fats, and high-quality protein foster beneficial probiotics to grow in the gut. Focusing on gut health is a vital part of managing cortisol symptoms.

KEY INSIGHT

The meal you eat for lunch is having a conversation with your stress hormones whether you're aware of it or not. Every food choice either signals safety or signals threat to your gut — and your cortisol responds accordingly.

Put your phone down at meals — here's why it matters for cortisol

Stop the relentless cortisol signaling, especially at mealtimes. This literally means putting your cell phone away, sitting in a comfortable place, slowly enjoying your food, keeping the television off, and avoiding any stressful conversations. Your body will absorb your food better and digest things better if you allow your nervous system to reset periodically throughout the day, especially at mealtimes.

When you eat in a stressed state — scrolling your phone, watching the news, or having a tense conversation — your body is in sympathetic (fight-or-flight) mode. Digestion is suppressed in this state. Nutrient absorption is impaired. The gut-brain axis interprets the meal as just another stress event rather than a recovery opportunity. Putting the phone down isn't a lifestyle suggestion. It's a physiological intervention.

The cortisol-free meal ritual

- Put the phone in another room or face-down
- Turn off the television and news
- Sit at a table rather than a desk or couch

- Take three slow breaths before your first bite
- Eat slowly enough to actually taste the food
- Avoid difficult conversations until 20 minutes after eating

These aren't rules — they're tools. Use what works. Even one or two consistently practiced will measurably improve digestion, nutrient absorption, and the cortisol response to your meal.

Include probiotic and prebiotic foods

Your gut bacteria have opinions about your stress levels. Strong ones. And the fastest way to get them back on your side is to feed them well and — when things have gone significantly sideways — reinforce them with the right supplements.

Fermented foods are the natural starting point. Yogurt, kefir, sauerkraut, kimchi, fermented vegetables — these aren't just trendy menu items, they're delivery vehicles for beneficial bacteria that actively improve brain function and protect neurons.[2] If you're not eating any of them regularly, that's the first easy change worth making.

Prebiotics — the fiber compounds in foods like onions, garlic, and bananas that feed your beneficial bacteria — are the supporting cast. Worth including, worth rotating, but with one important caveat: the research behind prebiotics is considerably less robust than the research behind **probiotics**, and for people with **IBS** or inflammatory bowel disease, certain prebiotic foods can cause more disruption than benefit. Listen to your gut here. Literally.

Now, the honest clinical observation from 26 years of watching people try both approaches: probiotic supplements consistently outperform fermented foods alone when it comes to measurable stress and cortisol reduction. This isn't a slight against sauerkraut. It's a numbers problem. The bacterial counts in encapsulated probiotics are significantly higher and more consistent than what most people actually eat day to day, and consistency is everything when you're trying to shift the gut microbiome. My clients who add a quality probiotic supplement to their routine almost universally notice a difference in how they feel — more so than dietary changes alone.

One important exception: if you have IBS, don't just grab whatever's on the shelf at the pharmacy. Certain probiotic strains can aggravate IBS symptoms rather than help them, and the wrong choice can set you back. This is one situation where a functional medicine practitioner is genuinely worth consulting before you start — getting the right strains for your specific situation makes a meaningful difference.

Avoid foods sprayed with glyphosate

As covered in Chapter 4, glyphosate isn't just an agricultural inconvenience — it directly disrupts **GABA**, the cortisol-balancing neurotransmitter, while simultaneously damaging the gut lining.[18] The practical problem is that it's sprayed on most conventionally grown grains and legumes — wheat, oats, corn, soy, beans, lentils, canola, and more — making avoidance genuinely tricky without some intention behind it.

The simplest solution: choose organic grains and legumes whenever possible. If organic isn't accessible or affordable, companies like Healthy Traditions sell verified glyphosate-free grain products worth knowing about.

Limit processed foods

Highly processed foods often contain many chemicals, additives, inflammatory fats, and high amounts of sugar that will negatively impact your gut health and have a negative effect on the cortisol response. If it comes in a package that's shinier than a neon sign, it's probably ultra-processed and bad for your mental health.

What your meal signals to your gut — and your cortisol

Ultra-processed meal fast food · packaged snacks · seed oils	**Cortisol-busting meal** salmon · roasted veg · sauerkraut · herbs
Gut alarm triggered	Happy gut bacteria activated
Inflammatory signals sent to brain	Serotonin produced in gut
Cortisol spike	Cortisol normalized
Nutrients depleted, cravings increase	Nutrients absorbed and restored
Loop worsens	**Healing cycle begins**

Two-column visual: Processed food meal versus cortisol-busting meal — showing gut signaling cascade each produces. Left: fast food burger → gut alarm → inflammatory signals → cortisol spike → nutrient depletion. Right: salmon + roasted vegetables + sauerkraut → happy gut bacteria → serotonin production → cortisol normalized → nutrients absorbed.

Include healthy fats

The healthy fat conversation is one of the most confused areas in all of nutrition — partly because the science has genuinely evolved, and partly because a lot of money has been spent making sure the wrong conclusions stuck around longer than they should have.

The oils to move away from

Seed oils — soybean, canola, corn, and their industrially processed cousins — are not the neutral cooking fats they're marketed as. They're heavily chemically processed, high in **linoleic acid** (a pro-inflammatory fat that research links to increased inflammatory disease),[9] and frequently contaminated with glyphosate residues from the growing process. The ubiquity of these oils in restaurant food, packaged snacks, and fast food means that simply eating out regularly puts you in contact with them constantly — which is worth knowing, even if you can't always avoid it.

Peanut oil and sunflower oil occupy a gray area. If you use them, organic and expeller-pressed versions are meaningfully cleaner, though glyphosate exposure in production remains a concern even then.

A note on cost and access

Switching away from seed oils is genuinely easier if you have a well-stocked grocery store nearby and a budget that allows for choices. Not everyone does, and it's worth saying plainly: if seed oils are what's available and affordable right now, that is a completely reasonable reality and not a personal failure. Do what you can with what you have. The goal is progress, not perfection.

Budget-friendly healthy fat swaps

- **Store-brand butter** instead of margarine or vegetable oil spreads
- **Olive oil** bought on sale and stored properly (away from heat and light)
- **Canned sardines or salmon** over expensive fresh fish — same omega-3s, fraction of the cost
- **Whole-fat plain yogurt** in large containers rather than individual flavored servings
- **Eggs** — one of the most nutrient-dense, affordable foods available

These are not compromises. They are genuinely good choices that happen to also be affordable.

The fats worth building meals around

Whole food fat sources are where the real nutritional value lives: fatty fish like salmon and sardines, extra-virgin olive oil, avocados, grass-fed meats, virgin coconut oil, nuts, seeds, and dairy — ideally grass-fed where budget allows, but conventional whole-fat dairy is still meaningfully better than low-fat processed alternatives. The goal is to include a healthy fat source at every meal, which helps stabilize blood sugar, support hormone production, and keep cortisol from spiking in response to the blood sugar crashes that fat-free eating tends to cause.

Coconut oil is worth singling out because it surprises people. Virgin coconut oil has shown improvement in memory in Alzheimer's patients[10] and meaningful reductions in anxiety and depression markers in animal studies.[11] It's also stable at high heat, which makes it a practical cooking fat.

Fish oil deserves its own mention. Multiple studies confirm that fish oil supplementation reduces baseline cortisol levels and dampens the stress response in the body.[7,8,20] If you're not eating fatty fish two to three times a week — and most people aren't — a fish oil supplement is one of the highest-value additions you can make. More on choosing one wisely in Chapter 6.

The saturated fat rehabilitation

Saturated fat has spent about forty years being treated as a nutritional villain, and the evidence for that characterization has quietly been falling apart. When the dietary guidelines began pushing Americans away from saturated fat in the 1980s, something had to replace those calories — and what replaced them, largely, was highly processed carbohydrates. The result was an American population that dutifully reduced saturated fat intake and proceeded to get significantly heavier, sicker, and more anxious. Heart disease rates, which the saturated fat restrictions were supposed to improve, have not meaningfully declined and by some measures continue to rise.[6]

Part of why this matters for cortisol specifically: cholesterol and saturated fat are essential raw materials for steroid hormone production — including cortisol itself, and the sex hormones that cortisol tends to deplete. A diet chronically low in these fats is a diet that makes hormone regulation harder, not easier.

Clinical research in overweight women found that higher dairy fat intake actually enhanced body fat loss while reducing cortisol production in belly fat tissue.[3] Whole-fat dairy also contains **butyrate**, a short-chain fatty acid that feeds and repairs the gut lining. The American Heart Association's continued insistence on limiting saturated fat is worth viewing with some skepticism, particularly given that the organization was founded with funding from Procter and Gamble — the makers of Crisco.[5] The most current review in the journal *Nutrients* found the evidence linking saturated fat to heart disease to be inconsistent and inconclusive at best.[4]

This doesn't mean eating saturated fat without any context. Butter on broccoli is a genuinely excellent choice — the fat supports nutrient absorption from the vegetables, the combination is satisfying, and there's nothing in it your body doesn't know how to use. Butter on a croissant made from refined flour, seed oils, and sugar is a different equation — not because of the butter, but because of everything surrounding it. Context matters. The fat is rarely the problem.

Plain whole-milk yogurt over sweetened low-fat yogurt. Butter over margarine. Salmon over a fat-free protein bar. These are not indulgences — they are the more nutritionally sound choices.

Stay hydrated

Adequate hydration aids in digestion and nutrient absorption. It also is critical for carrying signals through the body that promote a sense of calm. What this means from person to person is different — thirst is the best indicator of the need for hydration, so simply drink water or herbal tea when you are thirsty. Herbal teas in particular are a double win: they hydrate while delivering the cortisol-balancing compounds covered in Chapter 7.

Get high-quality protein

As a building block of hormones and signaling molecules, protein helps balance cortisol. Protein is also a major building block of gut cells, while also helping to fuel probiotics. Good protein sources include fish, grass-fed meats, bone broth, organic poultry, plain unsweetened Greek yogurt, and grass-fed whey protein. Some intriguing research shows that a higher-protein diet significantly reduces the risk of anxiety and depression.[17] The exact amount of protein that is ideal for you should be individualized, but it is clear that the RDI for protein is too low for optimizing lean muscle and mood.

Not all protein is equal

While legumes have some protein, be very careful to choose organic if you do choose to eat them. For example, tofu made from soybeans can contain very unsafe levels of glyphosate, which hinders gut function and thus increases the stress response. This could be part of why vegetarians struggle with higher rates of anxiety and depression.[12] And the volume of legumes it takes to get enough protein is substantial. For example, it takes 4 cups — or almost 2.5 pounds — of prepared refried beans to equal 48 grams of protein, while only 8 ounces of salmon gets you that same amount of protein. The protein quality score is also lower in legumes than it is in salmon.[19]

Not all protein is equal

To get 48g of protein for cortisol recovery — legumes vs. wild salmon

Category	Plant protein (refried beans)	Animal protein (wild salmon)
Quantity needed to reach 48g protein	4 cups / ~2.5 lbs high carbohydrate load	8 oz fillet lean, no extra carbs
Protein quality score (DIAAS / digestibility)	Lower incomplete amino acid profile	Higher complete amino acid profile
Chemical exposure glyphosate / pesticides	High risk if conventional disrupts GABA + gut lining	Minimal risk wild-caught is clean
Inflammation effect on cortisol loop	May trigger gut inflammation in sensitive individuals	Anti-inflammatory omega-3s directly reduce baseline cortisol
Preparation needed to reduce anti-nutrients	Soak, sprout, or cook to reduce phytates and lectins	Ready to cook highly bioavailable amino acids
Cortisol-specific nutrients provided	Magnesium, folate good if organic pair with taurine foods	Omega-3, B12, D3 zinc, selenium complete adrenal support

If choosing plant proteins: always buy organic · pair with taurine-rich foods for GABA support
Amino acids are the building blocks of the hormones and neurotransmitters that regulate cortisol

Amino acids, as building blocks of hormones and hormone receptors in the body, have very intriguing benefits for mental health and cortisol. I will review these further in Chapter 6. You should also try to get plenty of taurine-rich foods such as clams, oysters, scallops, dark meat turkey, and grass-fed meats or wild game. Taurine helps regulate **GABA**.[13]

Get GABA foods, spices, and herbs

GABA is an important compound in the body that helps balance out the effects of cortisol. There are several categories of foods that can help, primarily fermented dairy, organic green tea, taurine-rich protein foods as listed above, and herbs like the following, which I will discuss in Chapter 7.[14]

GABA-supporting foods at a glance

- **Fermented dairy** — kefir, yogurt, aged cheese (also supply probiotics)
- **Organic green tea** — L-theanine enhances GABA activity (see COMT gene note in Chapter 7)
- **Taurine-rich foods** — clams, oysters, scallops, dark meat turkey, grass-fed meats
- **Herbs with rosmarinic acid** — mint, lemon balm, rosemary, thyme, oregano, sage
- **Curcumol spices** — turmeric and ginger
- **Apigenin-rich herbs** — chamomile, celery, parsley, passionflower

Other tips to manage cortisol

- **Don't eat after dinner.** Eating late can disrupt sleep and throw cortisol out of balance.[21] Eating more of your calories earlier in the day and eating adequate protein and magnesium can help curb your cravings for sugar in the evening.
- **Increase certain fibers.** Foods high in certain dietary fibers, such as fruits, vegetables, and nuts, can support a healthy gut microbiome. But some people are very sensitive to fiber-rich foods, so be mindful of foods that cause your gut distress. Gut distress can make you stressed, and that's exactly what we are trying to avoid in this book! Healthy fiber sources include: hulled pumpkin seeds, chia seeds, sweet potatoes, gold potatoes, nuts and seeds, quinoa, beans, gluten-free oat bran, fruits, and vegetables. Choose organic because of the heavy chemical burden of conventionally grown foods.
- **Take high-quality vitamins and minerals.** Low levels of nutrients caused by stress can actually increase the risk of stress and trauma. For example, low levels of vitamin D increase the risk of PTSD. Incorporating a broad-spectrum natural multivitamin along with extra vitamin D may help increase the body's resilience to stress. I will review

vitamins, minerals, and other dietary supplements that are beneficial for stress in Chapter 6.

The power of food sensitivities

Our modern world is taking a serious toll on the gut. This is tragic because the gut is the gatekeeper for our bodies in a lot of ways. The increasing rates of food sensitivities and allergies are also contributing to elevated cortisol. They are a big driver of **inflammation**, and inflammation is one of the root causes of all chronic diseases. The reasons for an increase in these conditions have many layers: increased chemicals used in agriculture, increased gut-disrupting prescriptions, increased intake of processed foods, and more.[15,16]

If you are sensitive to a food, it isn't just miserable — it causes inflammation and imbalances in our immune responses. For example, gluten sensitivity can increase the chances of getting chronic diseases such as autoimmune diseases[15] and heart disease.[16] It also causes the body to feel like it's under threat, caused by immune system imbalances starting in the gut.

Food sensitivity testing can be challenging, but one test that has been very helpful for myself and my clients in determining their sensitivities is called the **Mediator Release Test** (MRT). This test measures the body's severity of inflammation in response to 176 foods and chemicals.[20] Other food sensitivity tests exist, such as IgG testing, but these tests are fraught with low sensitivity and specificity.

MRT testing can help people overcome migraines, inflammatory gut issues, skin issues, stress, and more. But you should always have a certified LEAP practitioner help guide you through this process. For more information, read about food sensitivity testing here: thehealthyrd.com/how-mrt-testing-transformed-my-health-from-the-inside-out

MRT vs. IgG food sensitivity testing

Why the test you choose matters — and what each one actually measures

Category	MRT Mediator Release Test	IgG testing standard antibody panel
What it measures	Actual inflammatory mediator release from white blood cells in response to foods	Antibody (IgG) levels — indicates exposure only, not inflammatory reaction
Question answered what is tested	Does your immune system react to this food? (reactive = symptomatic)	Have you been exposed to this food before? (exposure ≠ reaction)
Foods and chemicals tested	176 foods and food chemicals including additives and dyes	90-200 foods typically chemicals rarely included
Clinical reliability accuracy in practice	High sensitivity and specificity Results reflect actual symptoms clinically actionable	Significant false positives and false negatives common often misleading in practice
Guides which protocol	LEAP — personalized anti-inflammatory eating plan	Generic elimination diet often overly restrictive
Clinical recommendation	**Recommended** used in this practice	**Not recommended** unreliable for clinical use

MRT information and LEAP practitioners:
thehealthyrd.com/how-mrt-testing-transformed-my-health-from-the-inside-out

Chapter 5 summary

The close relationship between cortisol and our meals unveils a whole new dimension of understanding and managing stress. As we look into this relationship, we recognize the powerful role that our gut — our "second brain" — plays in both physical and mental health. People grappling with high cortisol are often navigating a maze of physical and psychological challenges. Our growing understanding of the gut-brain axis shines a light on the benefits of focusing on nutritional healing.

A balanced, nutrient-rich diet can contribute to a healthier cortisol response, offering many benefits for managing stress symptoms as reviewed above. By taking charge of your diet, you can actively engage in your own healing process, fostering not only improved gut health but also enhanced overall well-being and reduced stress.

However, it's crucial to remember that while nutritional interventions offer promising support, they are not standalone solutions. People with high levels of stress or PTSD should seek professional guidance to ensure their approach to managing their condition is comprehensive and tailored to their individual needs. A multi-pronged approach is always best.

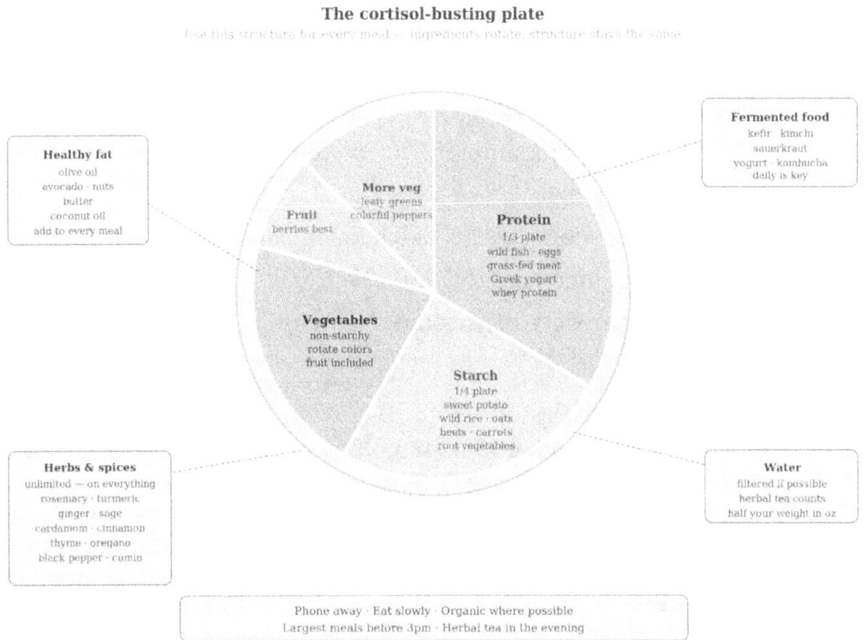

References

1 Gut microbiome and mealtime stress. *Nutrients*. 2020. https://pmc.ncbi.n lm.nih.gov/articles/PMC7442351/

2 Wang H, et al. Fermented foods and neuroprotection. *Nutrients*. 2016. https://pmc.ncbi.nlm.nih.gov/articles/PMC5216880/

3 Hadi A, et al. Dairy fat and cortisol production. *Eur J Nutr*. 2021. https://pmc.ncbi.nlm.nih.gov/articles/PMC3735906/

4 Astrup A, et al. Saturated fats and health: A reassessment. *J Am Coll*

Cardiol. 2020. https://pmc.ncbi.nlm.nih.gov/articles/PMC8541481/

5 Conflicts of interest in nutrition research. *Nutrients.* 2022. https://pmc.ncbi.nlm.nih.gov/articles/PMC9794145/

6 Heart disease rates rising. NHLBI. 2021. https://www.nhlbi.nih.gov/news/2021/cardiovascular-disease-rise-we-know-how-curb-it-weve-done-it

7 Barbadoro P, et al. Fish oil and cortisol. *Mol Nutr Food Res.* 2013. https://pubmed.ncbi.nlm.nih.gov/23390041/

8 Delarue J, et al. Fish oil and cortisol response. *Br J Nutr.* 2003. https://pubmed.ncbi.nlm.nih.gov/12909818/

9 Linoleic acid and inflammation. *J Nutr Biochem.* 2023. https://pubmed.ncbi.nlm.nih.gov/37400966/

10 Lima SM, et al. Coconut oil and Alzheimer's disease. *Nutrients.* 2024. https://pubmed.ncbi.nlm.nih.gov/37980665/

11 Coconut oil and anxiety/depression. *Nutrients.* 2024. https://pubmed.ncbi.nlm.nih.gov/34881837/

12 Food insecurity and depression in vegetarians. *Nutrients.* 2020. https://pubmed.ncbi.nlm.nih.gov/32483598/

13 Taurine and GABA. *Front Neurosci.* 2019. https://pmc.ncbi.nlm.nih.go v/articles/PMC6671153/

14 GABA-promoting foods. *Front Nutr.* 2021. https://pmc.ncbi.nlm.nih.g ov/articles/PMC7914492/

15 Gluten sensitivity and autoimmune disease. *Expert Rev Clin Immunol.* 2018. https://www.tandfonline.com/doi/full/10.1080/1744666X.2018.152 4757

16 Lebwohl B, et al. Celiac disease and heart disease. *BMJ.* 2017. https://w ww.bmj.com/content/357/bmj.j1892

17 Phillips SM, et al. Dietary protein and anxiety/depression. *Nutr Metab.* 2010. https://pubmed.ncbi.nlm.nih.gov/20849868/

18 Glyphosate and GABA disruption. *Toxicol Lett.* 2024. https://pubmed. ncbi.nlm.nih.gov/39401670/

19 Soy protein quality vs. salmon. *J Nutr.* 2022. https://jn.nutrition.org/ article/S0022-3166(22)14150-7/fulltext

20 MRT food sensitivity testing. *J Integr Med.* 2008. https://www.davidp

ublisher.com/Public/uploads/Contribute/5aa87a8e491ec.pdf

21 High calorie meals and cortisol reactivity. *Nutrients.* 2023. https://pmc.ncbi.nlm.nih.gov/articles/PMC10305480/

6

Chapter 6

UP YOUR CORTISOL-HEALING SUPPLEMENT GAME

Let me guess.

You've tried eating better. You've cut the sugar, added the vegetables, maybe even bought the expensive extra-virgin olive oil. You got a massage and listened to a meditation app on your phone. And you still feel exhausted, wired at midnight, soft around the middle, and vaguely like yourself from ten years ago has filed a missing persons report.

Here's what nobody told you: food alone can't fix this. Not because you're doing it wrong — but because chronic stress is metabolically expensive in a way that diet simply cannot keep up with. Your body is burning through nutrients faster than any plate of salmon and roasted vegetables can replace them. This isn't a personal failing. It's chemistry.

That's what this chapter is about.

KEY INSIGHT

If you are chronically stressed, virtually every vitamin and mineral in your body is running low. Not slightly low. Meaningfully, symptom-causingly low. Cortisol is expensive — it burns through magnesium, B vitamins, vitamin C, zinc, and vitamin D at a rate your diet genuinely cannot match.

I've spent years in the National Library of Medicine tracking down this research, and the picture it paints is consistent: stress creates deficiency, deficiency worsens stress, and the cycle continues until something interrupts it.

That something is what this chapter is about.

I want to be honest with you about something that might be uncomfortable. If you've been told by a doctor to stop taking supplements, you were given well-meaning advice from someone who almost certainly received fewer than 20 hours of nutrition training in medical school. That's not a criticism of your doctor as a person — most of them are working incredibly hard under impossible conditions. But "stop taking supplements" is the nutritional equivalent of telling someone with a broken leg to walk it off. It keeps people stuck, and I've watched it happen for decades.

If you only do three things

This chapter covers a lot of ground. If you're overwhelmed, start here and come back for the rest later.

Morning: Methylated B complex with breakfast. Make sure the label says "methylfolate" and "pyridoxal-5-phosphate" — if it says "folic acid" or "pyridoxine," put it back. Seeking Health and Thorne brands both fit the bill.

With a meal: Vitamin D3 (2,000–5,000 IU) with vitamin K2. Nearly everyone is deficient. It directly lowers the cortisol-to-cortisone ratio, supports mood, and costs almost nothing.

Before bed: Magnesium glycinate (300 mg). This single supplement improves sleep, reduces sugar cravings, calms the nervous system, and begins restoring what cortisol has been stealing from your bones and tissues for years. Most people notice a difference within a week.

Give these three a month. Then come back and read the rest of this chapter.

If you only do three things

The highest-impact supplements for cortisol management — start here

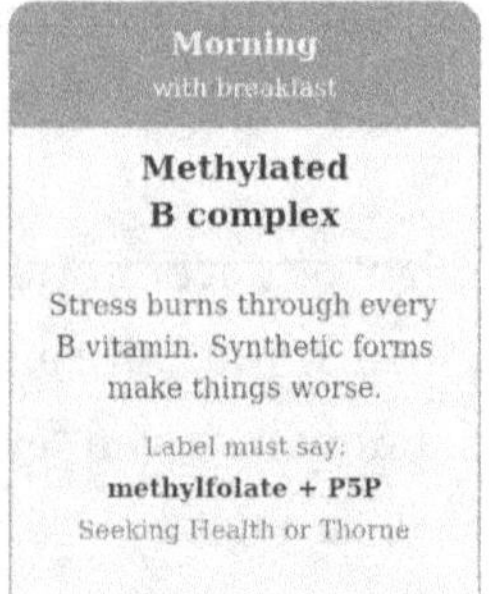

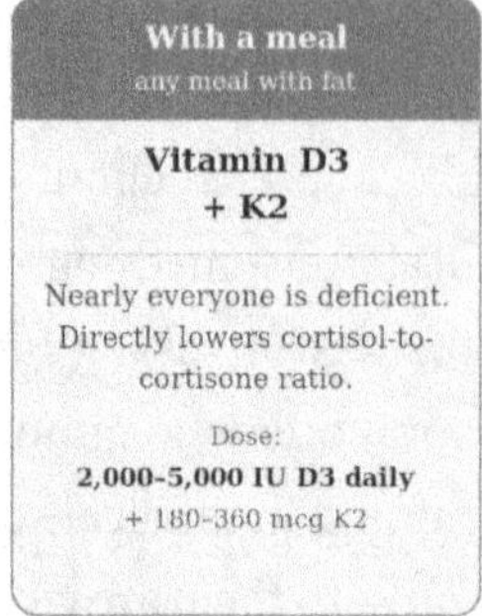

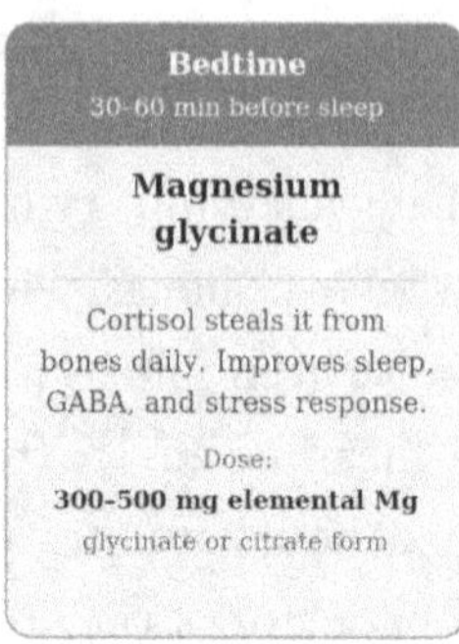

Give these three a month. Most people notice a difference within a week.
Then return to Chapter 6 to build from there.

Choosing high-quality supplements

Your supplements should come from reputable companies with third-party testing, known as certified Good Manufacturing Practices. Natural is always better, and I will teach you how to find natural versions of nutrients as we make our way through this chapter.

Some supplement manufacturers on major distribution sites can have fake or inferior products. Fullscript is a better alternative dispensary because all supplements sold there are third-party tested, pharmaceutical grade, and vetted by healthcare providers. Fullscript also does additional testing for purity and quality. For this reason, I suggest asking your healthcare provider who has a Fullscript account to recommend brands and doses. Alternatively, you can use my Fullscript account at https://us.fullscript.com/welcome/hm oretti. As full disclosure, I do make a small amount of affiliate income with this link.

You may want to gradually add supplements. A good rule of thumb is to start with a good B complex and magnesium, then add others one at a time. You'll find a full summary table at the end of this chapter.

Natural B vitamins visibly reduce high cortisol symptoms

You know that feeling where you're working but running on fumes — like some essential part of you has simply left the building? That's what B vitamin depletion feels like from the inside. Your body is running, but it's running on fumes, and the warning light has been on so long you've started to think it's decorative.

B vitamins are cortisol's favorite snack. Stress eats through them constantly, and then — in a move that feels almost personal — many of the medications prescribed for stress-related conditions deplete them further.[51] Metformin, birth control, blood pressure medications, GLP-1 drugs, stomach acid blockers: all of them quietly pick your B vitamin pockets while you're focused on other things.

The fix sounds simple: take a B complex. And it is simple, with one maddening catch. Most B complexes are synthetic. They look real, they're priced like they're real, they're sold at every pharmacy in America — and they can actually make things worse, particularly the fake versions of B6 and B12 that interfere with the very pathways you're trying to support.

You want a B complex that says *methylfolate, pyridoxal-5-phosphate*, and *methylcobalamin* on the label. If it says *folic acid, pyridoxine*, or *cyanocobalamin*, put it back and walk away.[7] The good stuff is in health food stores, functional medicine dispensaries, or from brands like Seeking Health or Thorne. Yes, it costs more. So does feeling terrible for another six months.

Personal account

I have watched clients' faces literally change within a week or two of switching to a quality methylated B complex. The puffiness around the eyes softens. The chinline looks more defined. The gray exhaustion lifts a little. They start handling Tuesday like Tuesday rather than like a personal affront.

Magnesium supplements make stress diminish

Here is a fun fact that is also deeply unfair: the more stressed you are, the more magnesium you lose. Which means the people who need it most are the ones losing it fastest. Cortisol essentially treats your magnesium stores the way a golden retriever treats an unattended sandwich — enthusiastically and without remorse.

Your bones have been quietly lending magnesium to the rest of your body for years to compensate. They are not happy about this. And because magnesium lives in your tissues rather than your blood, your doctor's blood test will read "normal" long after your actual stores have been quietly ransacked.[1] You can be depleted for a decade before it shows up on any lab work.

Take magnesium glycinate. Start with 300 mg at bedtime. Not magnesium oxide — that's the supplement equivalent of a knock-off handbag: technically the right shape, functionally disappointing. Glycinate absorbs well, relaxes muscles, improves sleep, and won't send you sprinting to the bathroom at 2am, which magnesium oxide cheerfully will. Citrate is also a great option and often cheaper than glycinate.

Using magnesium supplements has a lot of benefits. It helps reduce insulin resistance, decreases stress, and improves quality of sleep, while also helping reduce period pain, premenstrual syndrome, and postmenopausal symptoms. But magnesium isn't just for women. Magnesium helps your muscles function, keeps your heart healthy, and supports a balanced and focused brain. Some research even shows that higher magnesium intake is related to a reduction in aggression.[6] The world could use less aggression these days.

Magnesium helps regulate and balance neurotransmitters in the body that are needed for healthy sleep, including **GABA**, dopamine, serotonin, and even melatonin. A review of 7 clinical trials concluded that magnesium reduces anxiety symptoms.[3] Magnesium supplements improve sleep quality and melatonin levels in elderly people with primary insomnia.[4] Fascinatingly, cortisol levels were also reduced in this study, indicating that magnesium has a whole host of benefits beyond just sleep.

How does magnesium work to reduce cortisol? Magnesium promotes the activity of GABA and diminishes the stress response of cortisol.[2] It also helps enhance the **COMT gene**, which determines how we respond to worry and stress.[7]

Commonly prescribed medications that deplete magnesium include: diuretics, proton pump inhibitors, antacids, antibiotics, corticosteroids, antiviral medications, ACE inhibitors, breast cancer drugs, and stimulants like Ritalin and Adderall. Alcohol and sugar also cause the body to lose magnesium.

Personal account

As a dietitian of 26 years, I would like to think I could get enough magnesium in my diet. I eat servings of magnesium-rich foods every day — nuts and seeds, leafy greens, dark chocolate, seafood, quinoa, beans, avocados, and dairy. Not so. These foods sadly have diminishing amounts of magnesium as modern farming practices have caused soil levels to decline. Adding a magnesium supplement daily for many months made my response to stress improve tremendously, reduced menstrual discomfort, and kept bowel movements regular. We all are happier and healthier for it.

There is one exception: if you are in end-stage kidney failure, check with your doctor first.

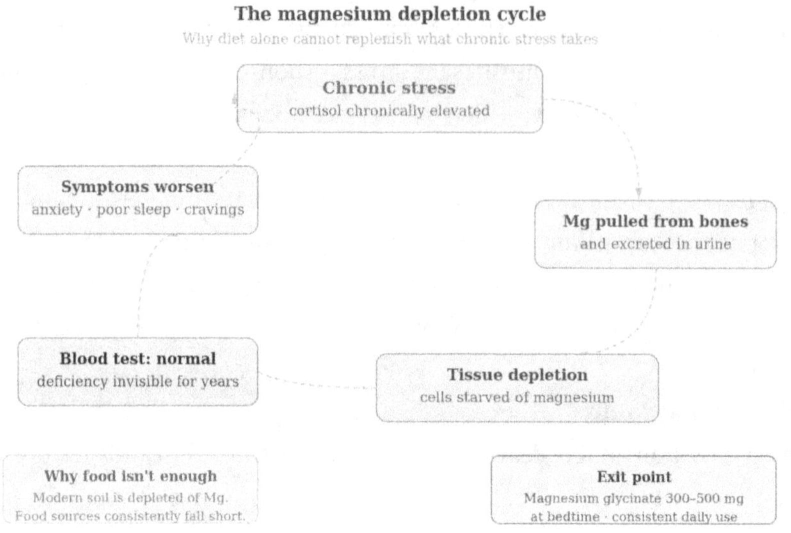

Diagram: The magnesium depletion-stress cycle — Chronic stress → cortisol spike → magnesium pulled from bones → tissue depletion → blood test reads normal → anxiety/poor sleep/sugar cravings worsen → more stress. Exit point: magnesium glycinate 300–500 mg at bedtime.

Vitamin C does more than prevent the common cold

Stress burns through vitamin C the way a fire burns through paper. Many clinical research trials have demonstrated the ability of vitamin C to decrease cortisol levels.[8] The government's official recommendation of 60 mg per day is enough to prevent scurvy — which is a low bar, and about as relevant to someone under chronic stress as a bicycle is to a fish. Research on cortisol reduction uses doses between 500 mg and 3,000 mg daily.[8] That gap is not a rounding error.

Using vitamin C supplements can be a very quick fix for reducing cortisol levels. Think of it like a rapid cortisol first-aid kit — keep some on hand in times of need. While there is some controversy around vitamin C and kidney stone risk, it appears to be a small increase in risk and only for men when using very high doses.[9] If you are male with a history of kidney stones, discuss this with your provider first.

One concern: most vitamin C supplements are synthesized from conventionally grown corn, which is produced with a heavy chemical burden. Look for whole-nutrient vitamin C without corn derivatives or synthetic ascorbic acid — brands like Premier Research Labs, Body Bio, or products using Quali-C® are reliable options. But any vitamin C is better than no vitamin C if you are on a budget.

Zinc is a healing nutrient for mood and immunity

Zinc doesn't get any respect. Overlooked and underestimated while vitamin D gets its own YouTube channel. Here's what zinc is actually doing while nobody's watching: regulating your immune response, directly reducing cortisol release from the adrenal glands, countering inflammation, supporting mood, and acting as an antioxidant throughout the whole operation. Low zinc levels are linked to anxiety in nine separate studies.[10] Nine. That's not a coincidence — that's a pattern.

Modern farming has stripped zinc from topsoil so efficiently that even people eating zinc-rich foods are often borderline deficient. If you're taking a proton pump inhibitor for heartburn, you are almost certainly low in zinc — these drugs block absorption so effectively that deficiency is nearly guaranteed with long-term use.[12]

Zinc supplementation reduces cortisol release from the adrenal glands directly.[11] Both physical and psychological stress cause people to lose more zinc, so stress in and of itself causes low levels. Zinc counters inflammation — another way it helps dampen the stress response. Researchers recently tracked 447 patients with inflammatory bowel disease and found 45.6% were zinc deficient.[13] The outcomes for zinc-deficient patients were dramatically worse across every measure: hospitalization, surgery, complications, and

ER visits.

The best food source of zinc is oysters, by a margin that isn't even close. After that: beef liver, crab, dark meat poultry, wild game. One genuine caution: don't take more than 50 mg daily long-term. High-dose zinc competes with copper for absorption, and trading one deficiency for another is not the goal.

Personal account

I keep zinc in my bag like other people keep Advil. When I take it at the first sign of illness, I feel better physically and mentally within minutes — and it's proven to do so. Just don't forget to take it with food.

Vitamin A to optimize cortisol and hormone sensitivity

Vitamin A has a resume problem. It was the very first vitamin ever discovered — literally vitamin number one, the one that started the whole category — and somehow it ended up as the quiet kid in the back of the nutritional classroom while vitamin D gets standing ovations and magnesium has its own wellness influencer pipeline.

When vitamin A runs low, cortisol overproduces.[15] Your thyroid goes sideways. Insulin resistance creeps in. Heavy periods worsen. Everything gets harder to manage — which, if you think about it, is exactly what happens to your car when you forget to change the oil.

The research is small but striking: vitamin A supplementation helped reduce cortisol even in people with Cushing's disease, which is essentially cortisol on its worst possible behavior.[16] If it can make a dent there, imagine what it does for the rest of us just trying to get through a Monday.

About 40% of people carry a gene variant that cripples their ability to convert plant-based vitamin A into the active form their body can use.[17] Forty percent. That's nearly half the room. All those people dutifully eating their carrots and sweet potatoes, feeling virtuous about their beta-carotene intake, and their bodies are essentially shrugging and filing it in the recycling bin.

Active vitamin A comes almost exclusively from animal sources. Liver is the undisputed champion. Cod liver oil is a strong second. Eggs contain some, but compared to liver they're bringing a knife to a gunfight. Fermented cod liver oil from Rosita or Green Pastures comes in gel caps — so no, you don't have to taste it. For vegetarians, vitamin A palmitate in supplement form is a reasonable option.

One note for pregnant readers: vitamin A is one of the few nutrients where excess genuinely matters during pregnancy. Run any supplementation by your provider before starting. For everyone else — the tolerable upper limit is 10,000 IU, short-term higher doses appear safe in research, and the risk of deficiency almost certainly outweighs the risk of modest supplementation for most people.[15,16,17]

Fish oil

Fish oil reduces baseline cortisol. Not just during stressful moments — your everyday starting point, lowered to more appropriate levels.[18] Multiple studies confirm that fish oil supplements are critical for reducing the stress response in the body.[18,19,20] Fish oil reduces stress levels in people who are recovering from alcoholism,[19] and the evidence across multiple populations is consistent.

To get the best fish oil supplements, choose fish oil in its triglyceride form and not its ethyl ester form. This can be difficult to find, but Nordic Naturals Ultimate Omega Fish Oil, Rosita cod liver oil, Now Tri 3-D fish oil, and Green Pastures cod liver oil are all in the correct form. Doses have a wide range — I encourage you to take the suggested dose on your supplement or discuss the optimal dose with your healthcare provider.

Limonene

You don't need a supplement for this one — you need a grater and a lemon or lime. Limonene is a potent nutraceutical derived from citrus peels of fruits like lemons, oranges, limes, fennel, and bergamot. It is also found in other plants like chamomile, ginger, rosemary, valerian, and cannabis. This antioxidant helps improve stomach health for many people by reducing acid reflux and indigestion symptoms.

According to early research, limonene helps improve GABA function in the brain[22] and has neuroprotective benefits, including protection from the toxicity of high cortisol.[23] A study of the ambient use of citrus essential oils in a dental clinic reduced anxiety and promoted calmness among people visiting the dentist.[21] Simply eating lemon, orange, and lime zest in cooking and in beverages is a safe, natural, and effective way to get limonene daily.

Amino acids that help heal the cortisol response

While many dietary supplements have improved my life and my clients' lives, the ones that continue to impress me most are amino acids. They are underused, yet can be highly effective for cortisol, depression, memory issues, and stress.

L-tyrosine for happy dopamine

Want to know what running low on dopamine feels like from the inside? Exactly like burnout. Dopamine, the happy-mood chemical, is directly made from L-tyrosine. L-tyrosine does a lot of other things too: it helps make thyroid hormone, improves energy, increases mental performance, reduces stress, and increases brain "flexibility" according to several early research studies.[24,25] Intense exercise robs the body of L-tyrosine.

The important balancing note: you should take L-tyrosine in a balanced ratio with L-tryptophan — a 10:1 ratio. A good example of an effective dose is 500 mg of L-tyrosine for every 50 mg of L-tryptophan. Taking too much without the balance may produce a headache or, rarely, increased anxiety symptoms. Start at the lowest dose and adjust from there.

L-tryptophan (5-HTP) for calming

Calm isn't just a feeling. It's a chemistry problem — and tryptophan is part of the solution. Research shows that 5-HTP acts to reduce symptoms of panic, a severe form of anxiety and cortisol response.[26] Tryptophan given before stressful situations reduces the hormonal and behavioral effects of stress.[26] A review of 11 clinical L-tryptophan studies concluded that it improves mood and emotional functioning.[27] This is because L-tryptophan is critical for making both melatonin and serotonin, and for managing cortisol.

Personal account

Several of my clients have tried a combination of L-tyrosine and 5-HTP and enjoy the brain benefits within minutes, not hours or weeks, as is the case for some prescription medications. The enhanced mood can last all day. Next time you feel a little off or blue, consider this a great tool to have in your toolbox. It works for me as well.

L-theanine for a calm vibe

Focused but not wired. Calm but not drowsy. That's what **L-theanine** does — and three separate clinical trials have now confirmed it. One study showed that L-theanine at 200 mg per day reduced anxiety symptoms, reduced depression symptoms, improved focus, and improved sleep quality.[29] A triple-blinded second study found very similar results.[30] A third study confirmed the effects, indicating that the results are real and not coincidental.[31]

Glycine: the warm blanket amino acid

Glycine reminds me of a warm blanket. It is comforting to the nervous system and gut. You may already be taking glycine without knowing it — it's the amino acid component of magnesium glycinate. Glycine helps to improve sleep quality by directly crossing the blood-brain barrier, where it works as a neurotransmitter.[32] It's helpful for promoting both falling asleep and deep sleep, and is likely helpful for mental health in many ways, including for OCD and other conditions like schizophrenia.

TMG (trimethylglycine) for enhancing mood

Originally discovered in beets, TMG — also known as betaine — is now showing up in research on cortisol, muscle performance, and mood. TMG enhances the production of SAMe, which helps with DNA maintenance, production of brain neurotransmitters, melatonin, and myelin. New research demonstrates that TMG reduces cortisol levels.[33] TMG also reduces post-exercise cortisol levels in athletes.[34] It is generally recognized as safe by the FDA.

Glutamine: muscle health while decreasing cortisol

Your immune cells run on glutamine the way your car runs on gas. Chronic stress drains the tank. Elevated cortisol in the body causes glutamine levels to plummet.[35] Several studies show that glutamine supplementation can reduce cortisol levels related to physical and mental stressors.[36] Glutamine supplementation even improves the ratio of testosterone to cortisol in athletes.[37] Supplemental glutamine can also help support weight loss by improving glucose metabolism — a review of 25 clinical studies concluded that glutamine does indeed help people with weight management.[36] Avoid glutamine if you are sensitive to MSG.

Vitamin D, calcium, and vitamin K2: not just for bone health

Almost everyone reading this book is deficient in vitamin D. Almost everyone. The ones who aren't are already supplementing or living close to the equator with regular sun exposure. Vitamin D is a critical hormone that helps regulate almost everything in the body. Vitamin D supplementation decreases the cortisol/cortisone ratio, which means it helps reduce the fight-or-flight response.[38] Supplemental vitamin D helps reduce cortisol levels overall in people with vitamin D deficiency.[39] This simple supplement reduces the risk of all major diseases.[40]

When stressed, your absorption of nutrients is reduced, including calcium. You also excrete more calcium under stress. This is where vitamin K2 comes in — it helps reduce the bone loss related to cortisol.[41] Make sure to take zinc and magnesium separately from calcium because they all compete for absorption in the gut, making none of them effectively absorbed when taken together.

Selenium for optimal adrenal function

Microplastics are accumulating in your body. Selenium helps clear them. That alone makes it worth paying attention to. Selenium is not only an essential nutrient — it is a potent antioxidant found in varying amounts in the soil where your food is grown. The best food source of selenium is Brazil nuts. I make a point to eat Brazil nuts daily throughout the cold and flu season.

Selenium supplementation may be beneficial for anxiety-related conditions, including prevention of anxiety following traumatic stress and obsessive-compulsive disorder.[42] Chronic stress reduces adrenal response, and low levels of selenium can contribute to a reduction in the production of balancing cortisone.[43] Selenium supplements may help recovery from adrenal fatigue[44] and reduce the microplastic burden in your body, which helps improve cortisol metabolism.[42] You should try to get between 100–200 mcg of selenium from food and/or supplements.

Iron deficiency causes cortisol burnout

Almost all of my women clients come to me iron deficient and fatigued as a result. Ten million Americans are low in iron.[48] Most of them don't know it. Many of them are being treated for anxiety instead. Iron deficiency increases your risk of anxiety — essentially excess cortisol.[45] If you are low in iron, your body's ability to make cortisol is impaired.[46] Other research indicates that optimizing iron levels in athletes may reduce cortisol levels.[47]

I'm a firm believer that each and every person should have their blood iron levels measured by testing transferrin saturation and ferritin. An ideal storage iron level, measured as ferritin, may be 70–100 ng/mL to maximize energy levels — this is considered above the normal range. But normal and optimal are two different things. If you have low iron levels, you can take iron supplements daily. Doses range between 20–65 mg per day, and I suggest re-checking your levels after 3–6 months.

Try coenzyme Q10 for physical and mental stress

If you are over thirty and under chronic stress, **CoQ10** is one supplement worth adding without much debate. Both physical and mental stress can deplete your body's CoQ10 reserves.[49] Women with polycystic ovarian syndrome who received CoQ10 supplementation experienced significantly less stress.[49] Similar results have been demonstrated in people with migraines and fibromyalgia.[49] This supplement has a high safety profile even at very high doses. More commonly, doses range between 100–400 mg per day.

Vitamin E reduces oxidative stress

Ninety percent of Americans don't get even the modest amount of vitamin E the government recommends. If you supplement vitamin E, you must absolutely make sure that you are using *natural* vitamin E and not synthetic. Look for supplements that contain natural tocopherols and natural tocotrienols to assure that you are not buying the inferior and potentially harmful synthetic version.[50]

Some of the best dietary sources of vitamin E are nuts, sesame seeds, chia seeds, poppy seeds, spices — particularly annatto and paprika — walnuts, pumpkin seeds, organic rice bran, and organic wheat germ (if you aren't sensitive to gluten). Vitamin E may help the adrenal gland work better because it helps lessen the production of stress-related chemicals like cortisol by fostering hormonal equilibrium.[50]

Supplement reference table

The following two tables consolidate all supplement information from this chapter. **Table 1** covers nutrients, benefits, and dosing. **Table 2** covers recommended brands and key considerations. Please pay close attention to the type of B vitamins you buy — they can be the most powerful for stress, but if you choose the wrong brands or forms, they can do more harm than good.

Chapter 6 supplement table — Table 1

Nutrients, key benefits, and amounts

Nutrient	Key benefits	Amounts
Natural B vitamins	Reduce cortisol; improve energy, metabolism, heart health, brain health	Varies by B vitamin type
Magnesium	Reduce cortisol; improve sleep, muscle function, digestive function, brain function	300–500 mg daily
Vitamin C	Reduces cortisol; natural antihistamine; supports immunity	500–1,000 mg, 1–3x daily
Zinc	Reduces cortisol; supports immunity; antioxidant	7–50 mg per day
Vitamin A	Improves cortisol and hormone sensitivity	Up to 10,000 IU; varies
Fish oil	Reduces stress and cortisol levels	1,000–3,000 mg daily
Limonene	Improves GABA function; neuroprotective	1,000 mg daily
L-Tyrosine	Improves energy, mental performance, reduces stress	250–1,000 mg; start low
L-Tryptophan (5-HTP)	Improves mood; builds melatonin and serotonin	25–100 mg daily
L-Theanine	Reduces anxiety and depression; improves focus and sleep	100–200 mg daily
TMG (Trimethylglycine)	Methyl donor; reduces cortisol; supports mood	500–1,000 mg daily
Glutamine	Stress depletes it; supplementation reduces cortisol	500–5,000 mg daily
Vitamin D3	Decreases cortisol/cortisone ratio	2,000–10,000 IU daily
Vitamin K2	Reduces bone loss from cortisol	180–360 mcg daily
Calcium	Improves bone density under chronic stress	500–1,000 mg if needed
Selenium	Reduces microplastic burden; dampens inflammation	100–200 mcg daily
Iron	Deficiency increases anxiety and cortisol	15–65 mg (test first)
Coenzyme Q10	Reduces oxidative stress from physical/mental stress	100–400 mg daily
Vitamin E	Reduces oxidative stress; supports adrenal function	100–400 IU daily

Chapter 6 supplement table — Table 2
Recommended brands and clinical considerations

Nutrient	Recommended brands	Considerations
Natural B vitamins	Seeking Health B Complex Plus; Thorne B vitamins	Must include methylfolate, P5P, methylcobalamin. Avoid folic acid, pyridoxine, cyanocobalamin.
Magnesium	Many brands	Best forms: glycinate, malate, or citrate. Avoid oxide. Use powders, gummies, or capsules; avoid tablets.
Vitamin C	Premier Research Labs; Body Bio; Quali-C® brands	Limit high doses if male with kidney stone history.
Zinc	Many brands	Zinc citrate, carnosine, glycinate are good forms. Avoid tablets.
Vitamin A	Rosita or Green Pastures cod liver oil; MK Supplements beef liver; Now vitamin A palmitate	Safe upper limit 10,000 IU; avoid in pregnancy without guidance.
Fish oil	Nordic Naturals Ultimate Omega; Rosita or Green Pastures cod liver oil; Now	Choose triglyceride form, not ethyl ester. Cod liver oil often superior.
Limonene	Integrative Therapeutics; Swanson	Easy to get from organic citrus rind.
L-Tyrosine	Brain MD	Take with tryptophan at 10:1 ratio (e.g. 500 mg tyrosine : 50 mg tryptophan).
L-Tryptophan (5-HTP)	Brain MD	Balance with tyrosine at 10:1 ratio.
L-Theanine	Pure Encapsulations; Now; Integrative Therapeutics	Occasionally causes headaches or nausea.
TMG	Life Extension; Brain MD	May not be needed if B vitamins are optimized.
Glutamine	Designs for Health; Pure Encapsulations	Best in powder form, sipped slowly. Avoid if sensitive to MSG.
Vitamin D3	Many brands	Take with meal. Combine with vitamin A, magnesium, K2, calcium, boron.
Vitamin K2	Many brands	Take with vitamin D3 cofactors.
Calcium	Many brands	Calcium citrate preferred. Take separately from iron, zinc, magnesium.
Selenium	Many brands	Selenomethionine and Se-Methyl L-Selenocysteine are best forms.
Iron	Many brands	Use only if ferritin/transferrin saturation is low. Optimal ferritin ~50 ng/dL.
Coenzyme Q10	Many brands	High safety profile.
Vitamin E	Many brands	Natural forms only: mixed tocopherols with tocotrienols.

Supplement timing guide

When to take each supplement for maximum cortisol benefit

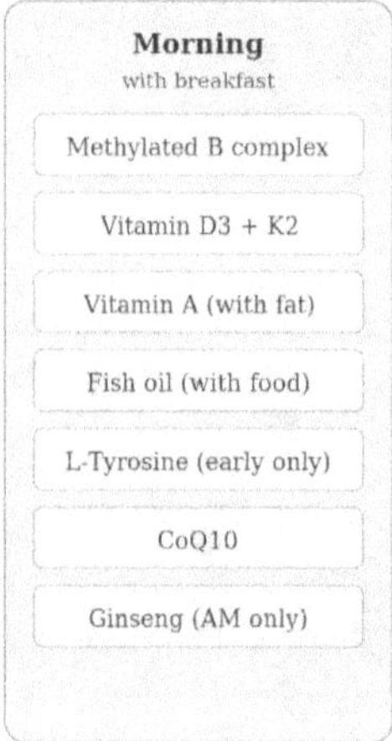

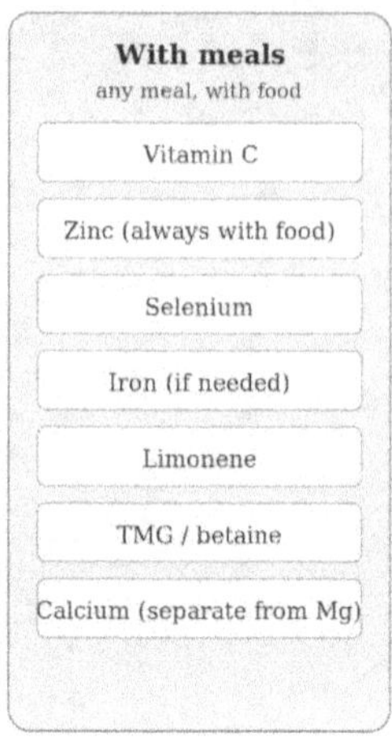

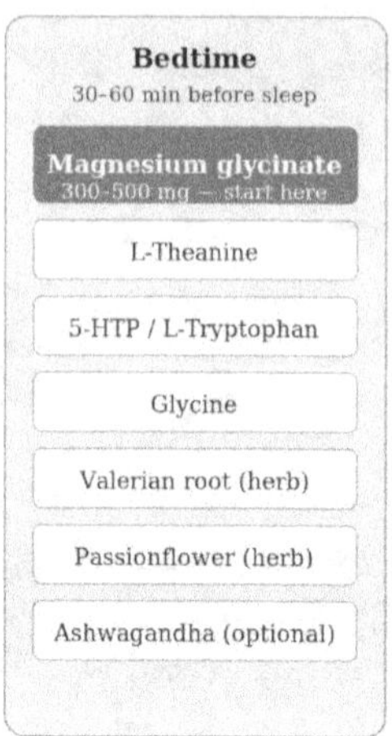

Separate calcium from magnesium, zinc, and iron — they compete for absorption

References

1 Pickering G, et al. Magnesium status and stress. Nutrients. 2020. https://www.mdpi.com/2072-6643/12/12/3672

2 Magnesium and stress. Nutrients. 2021. https://pmc.ncbi.nlm.nih.gov/articles/PMC7761127/

3 Botturi A, et al. Magnesium in mental disorders. Nutrients. 2020. https://www.sciencedirect.com/science/article/pii/S0149763423001288

4 Magnesium and mental health overview. Nutrients. 2023. https://pmc.ncbi.nlm.nih.gov/articles/PMC10255717/

5 Limbourg A, et al. Magnesium in soil and food supply. Front Plant Sci. 2020. https://pmc.ncbi.nlm.nih.gov/articles/PMC7649274/

6 Magnesium and aggression. Front Nutr. 2021. https://pmc.ncbi.nlm.nih.gov/articles/PMC8098670/

7 COMT gene and mental health. MyGenefood. https://www.mygenefood.com/genes/brain-and-mental-health-genes/comt/

8 Carr AC, et al. Vitamin C and cortisol. Nutrients. 2020. https://pmc.nc
bi.nlm.nih.gov/articles/PMC7024758/

9 Taylor EN, et al. Vitamin C and kidney stones. J Urol. 2016. https://pm
c.ncbi.nlm.nih.gov/articles/PMC4769668/

10 Zinc and anxiety: systematic review. J Affect Disord. 2023. https://pu
bmed.ncbi.nlm.nih.gov/37364014/

11 Zinc and cortisol from adrenal glands. Biol Trace Elem Res. 1998.
https://link.springer.com/article/10.1007/BF02789143

12 PPI and anxiety/depression risk. J Psychosom Res. 2023. https://pub
med.ncbi.nlm.nih.gov/35015332/

13 Zinc deficiency in IBD. Nutrients. 2025. https://www.mdpi.com/207
2-6643/17/21/3378

14 Zinc and phytates in plant-based diets. Am J Clin Nutr. 2013. https://p
mc.ncbi.nlm.nih.gov/articles/PMC3724376/

15 Vitamin A and cortisol production. Biochim Biophys Acta. 2014.
https://pmc.ncbi.nlm.nih.gov/articles/PMC3912436/

16 Vitamin A and Cushing's disease. Eur J Endocrinol. 2019. https://pub
med.ncbi.nlm.nih.gov/29881371/

17 BCMO1 gene and vitamin A conversion. ScienceDaily. 2016. https://w
ww.sciencedaily.com/releases/2016/12/161207124055.htm

18 Barbadoro P, et al. Fish oil and cortisol. Mol Nutr Food Res. 2013.
https://pubmed.ncbi.nlm.nih.gov/23390041/

19 Delarue J, et al. Fish oil and cortisol response. Br J Nutr. 2003. https://p
ubmed.ncbi.nlm.nih.gov/12909818/

20 Fish oil and cortisol. Nutrients. 2021. https://pmc.ncbi.nlm.nih.gov/a
rticles/PMC8510994/

21 Limonene aromatherapy and anxiety. Phytomedicine. 2001. https://p
ubmed.ncbi.nlm.nih.gov/11134689/

22 Limonene and GABA. J Agric Food Chem. 2021. https://pubmed.ncbi.
nlm.nih.gov/33548867/

23 Limonene neuroprotection. Biomed Pharmacother. 2019. https://pub
med.ncbi.nlm.nih.gov/31103492/

24 L-tyrosine and stress. Physiol Behav. 1989. https://pubmed.ncbi.nlm.

nih.gov/2736402/

25 L-tyrosine and brain function. Nutrients. 2024. https://pubmed.ncbi.nlm.nih.gov/38975711/

26 L-tryptophan and cortisol. Nutrients. 2020. https://pubmed.ncbi.nlm.nih.gov/32272859/

27 L-tryptophan and mood. Nutrients. 2022. https://pubmed.ncbi.nlm.nih.gov/22717170/

28 L-tryptophan and sense of control. Psychopharmacology. 2005. https://pubmed.ncbi.nlm.nih.gov/15691531/

29 L-theanine and anxiety. Nutrients. 2019. https://pmc.ncbi.nlm.nih.gov/articles/PMC6836118/

30 L-theanine triple-blinded study. J Am Coll Nutr. 2021. https://pubmed.ncbi.nlm.nih.gov/34562208/

31 L-theanine and stress. Nutrients. 2024. https://pubmed.ncbi.nlm.nih.gov/38758503/

32 Glycine and sleep. J Pharmacol Sci. 1994. https://pubmed.ncbi.nlm.nih.gov/7980477/

33 TMG and cortisol. Patsnap Eureka. https://eureka.patsnap.com/report-measuring-the-role-of-trimethylglycine-in-stress-hormone-regulation

34 TMG and post-exercise cortisol. J Int Soc Sports Nutr. 2022. https://pubmed.ncbi.nlm.nih.gov/35599921/

35 Glutamine and cortisol. Amino Acids. 1990. https://pubmed.ncbi.nlm.nih.gov/3048115/

36 Glutamine supplementation and cortisol. Nutrients. 2017. https://pubmed.ncbi.nlm.nih.gov/28272402/

37 Glutamine and testosterone:cortisol ratio. Nutrients. 2024. https://pmc.ncbi.nlm.nih.gov/articles/PMC10783826/

38 Vitamin D and cortisol:cortisone ratio. Front Endocrinol. 2016. https://pmc.ncbi.nlm.nih.gov/articles/PMC4973406/

39 Vitamin D supplementation and cortisol. Int J Endocrinol. 2020. https://pubmed.ncbi.nlm.nih.gov/31957555/

40 Vitamin D and all-cause mortality. J Clin Endocrinol Metab. 2024. https://pubmed.ncbi.nlm.nih.gov/38824035/

41 Vitamin K2 and cortisol-related bone loss. Front Endocrinol. 2018. https://www.frontiersin.org/journals/endocrinology/articles/10.3389/fendo.2018.00526/full

42 Selenium and anxiety. Future Pharmacol. 2022. https://www.mdpi.com/2673-9879/2/4/37

43 Selenium and cortisone production. J Endocrinol. 2004. https://pubmed.ncbi.nlm.nih.gov/15322334/

44 Selenium and adrenal fatigue. J Endocrinol. 2014. https://pubmed.ncbi.nlm.nih.gov/24437222/

45 Iron deficiency and anxiety. BMC Psychiatry. 2013. https://bmcpsychiatry.biomedcentral.com/articles/10.1186/1471-244X-13-161

46 Iron and cortisol production. Am J Clin Nutr. 1991. https://pubmed.ncbi.nlm.nih.gov/1651678/

47 Iron and cortisol in athletes. Nutrients. 2019. https://pubmed.ncbi.nlm.nih.gov/30818782/

48 Prevalence of iron deficiency. Am J Clin Nutr. 2013. https://pmc.ncbi.nlm.nih.gov/articles/PMC3685880/

49 CoQ10 and stress. Front Endocrinol. 2020. https://pmc.ncbi.nlm.nih.gov/articles/PMC7730520/

50 Vitamin E and adrenal function. Antioxidants. 2023. https://pmc.ncbi.nlm.nih.gov/articles/PMC9824658/

51 Medication depletion of B vitamins. Nutrients. 2018. https://pmc.ncbi.nlm.nih.gov/articles/PMC6109862/

7

Chapter 7

CHAPTER 7

PLANT MEDICINES THAT EFFECTIVELY MANAGE CORTISOL

Long before there were clinical trials, there were gardens. And before there were gardens, there were people walking through forests and fields paying close attention to what happened when they ate or smelled or brewed certain plants. The knowledge they accumulated over thousands of years — passed through cultures, refined by observation, embedded in traditions on every continent — is the foundation this chapter is built on.

Modern research is catching up to a lot of it. Not all of it, and not fast enough — partly because plants can't be patented and therefore don't attract pharmaceutical funding. But the herbs in this chapter have enough research behind them to be taken seriously, and enough traditional history behind them to suggest the research is confirming something real rather than discovering it for the first time.

This is the longest chapter in the book for good reason: there are a lot of genuinely useful plants, and you deserve to know about them. You don't need all of them. Most people benefit enormously from two or three used consistently. Use the roadmap graphic below and the symptom clusters to find your starting point, then come back for the rest when you're ready.

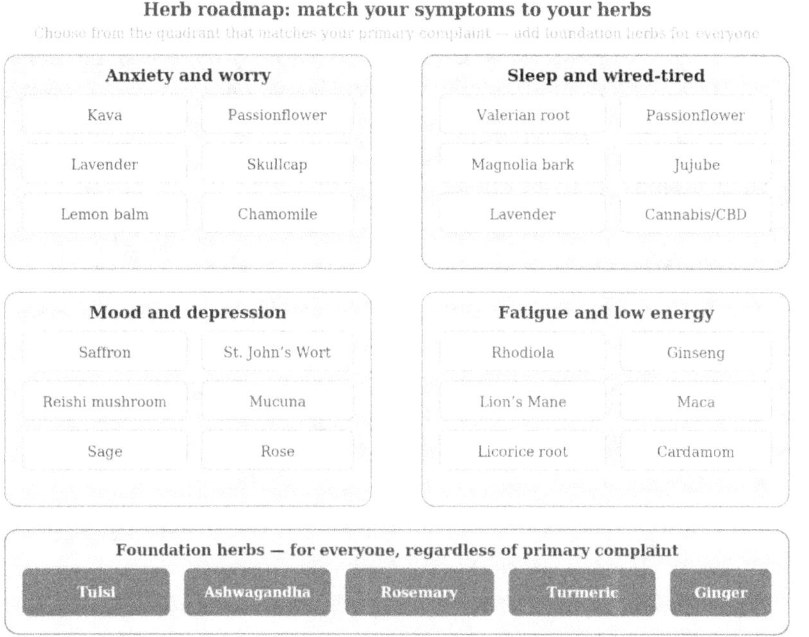

Herb roadmap: Four symptom clusters — Anxiety & stress (Ashwagandha, Lavender, Chamomile, Lemon balm); Sleep (Valerian, Passionflower, Kava, Magnolia bark); Mood & depression (Saffron, Rhodiola, Tulsi, Rose); Energy & focus (Lion's Mane, Ginseng, Rosemary, Green tea). Foundation row: Magnesium glycinate at bedtime + Methylated B complex with breakfast. Footer: Some herbs take 2–4 weeks. Start one at a time. Check with provider if pregnant or on medications.

How to choose quality natural plant medicines

The herb market has the same quality problem as the supplement market: some products are excellent, some are adequately mediocre, and some are barely what they claim to be on the label. Unlike pharmaceuticals, herbal products don't require pre-market approval by the FDA — which means the burden of quality assessment falls on you and, ideally, on a knowledgeable practitioner helping to guide your choices.

A few principles that hold up across the board:

- **Standardized extracts** matter for clinical herbs like ashwagandha, rhodiola, and ginseng. Look for the standardization percentage on the label (e.g., KSM-66 ashwagandha standardized to 5% withanolides). This tells you the active compound content is controlled and consistent.
- **Organic certification** matters most for herbs used at high doses or daily over the long term. Conventionally grown herbs can carry pesticide residues that work directly against the cortisol goals you're trying to achieve.
- **Third-party testing** — NSF Certified for Sport, USP, or ConsumerLab verified — adds meaningful assurance that what's on the label is actually in the bottle.
- **Fullscript dispensary** (us.fullscript.com/welcome/hmoretti) carries only third-party tested, pharmaceutical-grade products vetted by health-care providers. All brands recommended in this chapter are either available there or come with a quality rationale.

Learning to observe plants

You don't need a medical license for this — just a nose and a willingness to make weird tea.

One of the things that has gotten genuinely lost in modern medicine's insistence on randomized controlled trials is the art of clinical observation. Hippocrates was prescribing celery for nervous disorders around 400 BC. He didn't have a phase III trial to cite. He had eyes, a nose, and several thousand patients. That kind of careful observation — sustained, systematic, honest about outcomes — produced knowledge that modern research is still catching up to.

I encourage you to develop your own version of this. Pay attention to how you feel when you eat or smell or brew different herbs. Keep simple notes if it helps. Notice whether your sleep changes, whether your stress response feels different, whether anything shifts. You are not a passive recipient of the research in this chapter — you are the most important experiment in your own health story, and your observations matter.

Do people have herbal deficiencies?

Here is a question worth sitting with: if the standard human diet for most of human history included diverse wild plants, bitter greens, aromatic herbs, and fermented foods — and the modern diet largely does not — is it possible that some of what we call "anxiety" or "chronic stress" is partly a deficiency in the compounds these plants provide?

I think the answer is yes. Not entirely, not in every case — but the GABA-enhancing, adaptogenic, anti-inflammatory compounds in the herbs in this chapter are not extras. They are part of what a human nervous system was designed to have available. When they're absent from the diet, the system runs without them. And a nervous system running without its natural regulators looks a lot like modern life.

Herb entries A–Z

Ashwagandha — *the heavy hitter*

Ashwagandha is the adaptogen that most people have actually heard of, which is either a sign that it's been successfully marketed or that it's genuinely that effective. I'd argue both, but the research is substantial enough that the marketing is warranted.

Multiple randomized controlled trials have demonstrated that ashwagandha reduces cortisol by up to 30%.[3] It also reduces anxiety, improves sleep quality, supports thyroid function, and has a safety profile clean enough that it's one of the first adaptogens I recommend to clients new to herbal medicine. A meta-analysis of clinical trials confirmed consistent benefits for stress and anxiety across populations.[3]

The active compounds are called withanolides, and standardization matters here more than with most herbs — look for KSM-66 or Sensoril on the label, both of which are well-researched forms with consistent withanolide content. Generic ashwagandha from non-standardized sources is pharmacologically unpredictable.

One practical note: ashwagandha can interact with thyroid medications and should be discussed with your provider if you're on levothyroxine or similar. It's not contraindicated, but the interaction is worth managing consciously.

Black cumin seed — *not the cumin in your taco seasoning*

First, a clarification worth making upfront: black cumin seed (*Nigella sativa*) — also called black caraway or kalonji — is an entirely different plant from the common cumin used in Mexican and Latin American cooking. They share a name and a general pungency, but that's where the similarity ends. Black cumin seed has been a staple of Middle Eastern and Indian cuisines for thousands of years, used simultaneously as a culinary spice and a medicinal one.

Its active compound, thymoquinone, is responsible for most of the documented benefits: reduced inflammation, improved blood pressure, better heart and lung function, and meaningful reductions in anxiety symptoms — all shown across multiple animal and human studies, and notably without significant side effects.[4]

The cortisol research is particularly compelling. A landmark randomized, double-blind, placebo-controlled trial found that 200mg of black cumin seed oil daily for 90 days substantially reduced cortisol levels, reduced stress, and increased melatonin.[4] Animal research also shows it increases GABA activity. File that under evidence worth taking seriously.

Personal account

I've supplemented black cumin seed oil for years and noticed a distinct quality difference from brand to brand. After trying several, I've settled on Now brand for its consistency. No financial relationship with them — just a long track record of it actually working.

Cannabis — *worth an honest conversation*

Cannabis is not for everyone, and it's not a first-line recommendation for most people reading this book. But for some people — particularly those dealing with significant anxiety, chronic pain, or PTSD — it has genuine therapeutic value that deserves an honest discussion rather than either reflexive enthusiasm or reflexive dismissal.

The research on CBD specifically is reasonably solid. Several studies show that low-dose CBD meaningfully reduces stress and anxiety,[5,6] with anti-inflammatory and pain-relieving effects as additional benefits. For sleep specifically, cannabis shows consistent benefit,[9] which matters for cortisol management given how directly poor sleep drives cortisol dysregulation the following day.

For PTSD, the observational evidence is encouraging,[7,8] and I've seen this play out with clients firsthand. It doesn't work for everyone with trauma history, but for some people it's one of the more effective tools available for managing a genuinely difficult condition.

- **Start with full-spectrum CBD oil** at 5–10mg per day and increase slowly. Full-spectrum products contain the full range of plant compounds, which tend to work more effectively together than isolated CBD alone.
- **Strain variation is real and significant.** There are hundreds of cannabis varieties with meaningfully different effects. Dispensary staff guidance is genuinely useful here.

- **The research landscape is messier than it should be.** Cannabis's legal status has created significant research bias in both directions. Interpret the literature with that in mind.

For real-world accounts of therapeutic cannabis use, Cannabis Health Radio is worth your time: cannabishealthradio.com.

Cardamom — *the spice your nervous system has been waiting for*

Cardamom is one of those spices that most people encounter exclusively in chai tea or Indian desserts and never think about again. Which is a shame, because it turns out to be doing considerably more than adding warmth to your latte.

Cardamom has been used in Ayurvedic and traditional Chinese medicine for centuries — primarily for digestive complaints, but also for calming the mind and easing anxiety. A 2023 meta-analysis of randomized controlled trials — eight studies, 769 participants, intervention periods of 8 to 16 weeks — found that cardamom supplementation at 3,000mg of green cardamom daily significantly reduced inflammatory markers, lowered blood pressure, and decreased cortisol levels.[10] For a kitchen spice, that's a meaningful result.

The practical application is genuinely simple. Add half a teaspoon of ground cardamom to your morning coffee or tea — it pairs especially well with both, softening the edge of caffeine while adding its own calming quality. At 3,000mg — the dose used in the research — you're looking at roughly one teaspoon of ground cardamom daily, easy to distribute across meals and drinks.

One of the more underrated spices in this chapter. Worth making a regular habit.

Celery — *it's an herb, not a diet food*

Celery has a reputation problem. For most people it exists primarily as a vehicle for peanut butter or a guilt-free snack that tastes like crunchy water. This undersells it considerably. Celery is botanically an herb, and its seeds and leaves in particular are dense with compounds that do genuinely interesting things for the nervous system.

The most significant is apigenin — the same flavone that activates benzodiazepine receptors and enhances GABA transmission.[42] In celery, apigenin also stimulates nerve growth in adults, which classifies it as a nootropic. Hippocrates was prescribing celery for nerve disorders around 400 BC, which — given what we now know about apigenin's receptor activity — turns out to have been a well-reasoned clinical call.

Beyond apigenin, celery contains bioflavonoids that help prevent excess cortisol production, magnesium for nervous system calm, and a compound called 3-n-butylphthalide that early research links to neurological conditions including Alzheimer's disease, Parkinson's disease, anxiety, depression, and epilepsy.[42] That's a lot of pharmacological activity from something most people think of as a garnish. Safety profile is essentially unlimited for most people — the one exception is severe kidney disease.

Personal account

I've used celery in various forms for years, but adding celery seed extract as a daily tincture has been one of the more noticeable recent changes to my own routine. Within a relatively short period, my mood improved measurably and my inflammation markers dropped. My joint and muscle comfort now genuinely feels like a decade younger — and I don't say that lightly. One dropperful of celery seed extract tincture stirred into water in the morning. Easy, inexpensive, and — based on both the research and my own experience — worth adding to the rotation.

Chamomile — *ancient, unglamorous, and quietly remarkable*

Chamomile is the herb that gets no respect. It sits in the back of the tea cabinet behind the exciting options, gets dismissed as something grandmothers drink, and has spent thousands of years being genuinely effective while everyone waited for something more impressive to come along.

Nothing more impressive has come along.

Clinical research confirms what traditional medicine has known for millennia: chamomile meaningfully reduces anxiety symptoms, outperforming placebo in controlled trials and showing particular effectiveness in people with moderate-to-severe generalized anxiety disorder.[11] It improves sleep quality, reduces depression symptoms, and begins working almost immediately rather than requiring weeks of loading before you notice anything.[11]

The practical dose from the research works out to roughly three cups of chamomile tea per day. By reducing cortisol and anxiety, chamomile also reduces stress-driven food cravings and the weight gain that tends to follow them — an herb that calms your nervous system, improves your sleep, lifts your mood, and quietly helps your waistline, with no meaningful side effects.

The pharmaceutical industry would charge a great deal of money for that profile. Chamomile costs about four dollars a box. Side benefits instead of side effects.

Feverfew — *the daisy that pulls its weight*

Feverfew looks like a cheerful wildflower. It has small white daisy-like blooms, grows easily, and seems entirely too pretty to be doing anything serious. Don't be fooled. This is one of the harder-working herbs in the chapter.

Traditionally used across multiple cultures for migraines, fevers, rheumatoid arthritis, digestive complaints, and muscle spasms, feverfew has a therapeutic range that most single herbs can't match.[13] Through its apigenin content, it works on GABA receptors in the same way chamomile does, helping balance the stress response and reduce cortisol symptoms.[13] If chamomile is the gentle option for anxiety and sleep, feverfew is the one you reach for when anxiety comes with a headache, joint pain, or muscle tension attached.

The migraine research is particularly well-established. Multiple trials confirm that feverfew reduces both the frequency and severity of migraines — not by suppressing pain after the fact, but by reducing the inflammatory cascade that triggers them.[14] For people whose stress reliably shows up as headaches, this is worth knowing.

Two practical notes: don't chew the raw leaves directly — long-term contact can cause mouth irritation. Teas, tinctures, and capsules don't cause this. And feverfew belongs to the daisy family — if you have sensitivities to chamomile, calendula, or ragweed, approach it cautiously.

Ginseng (Panax) — *the adaptogen that actually gives you energy*

Ginseng has been used in traditional medicine for thousands of years, which means it has also been used in approximately ten thousand wellness products of wildly varying quality and effectiveness. Setting aside the ginseng-flavored energy drinks and the dubious capsules at gas station checkout counters, the actual root — specifically Panax ginseng, the Korean or Asian variety — is one of the more thoroughly researched adaptogens available.

In men with metabolic syndrome, ginseng increases testosterone while reducing cortisol.[21] In stressed adults generally, it improves mood, reduces anxiety, and measurably improves brain function compared to placebo.[21] The cognitive effects are notably fast: performance improvements documented at one hour, three hours, and six hours after a single dose — consistent across three separate clinical reviews.[22]

A preliminary study found ginseng performed comparably to diazepam (prescription Valium) for anxiety relief, without the sedation, dependency risk, or withdrawal effects. The mechanism involves GABA and serotonin enhancement alongside nootropic effects on nerve growth.[23]

Important nomenclature note: Panax ginseng (Korean or red ginseng) has the strongest research support. American ginseng hasn't been tested to the same standard. Indian ginseng is ashwagandha, an entirely different plant. Verify Panax ginseng specifically on the label when buying. And because ginseng is stimulating in a way that most calming herbs are not, take it in the morning. This is not a bedtime tea.

Green tea — *energizing, relaxing, and more complicated than it looks*

Green tea occupies a unique pharmacological space: it's simultaneously stimulating and calming, which sounds contradictory until you understand that caffeine and **L-theanine** — both present in green tea — work on different neurological pathways and balance each other out in ways that coffee simply doesn't. A review of four clinical studies confirms: it reduces anxiety symptoms while improving memory and focus.[18] Quality varies enormously. Organic matcha is worth the upgrade — higher catechin content and considerably more of the compounds that make the research results possible.

The worry gene — and why green tea makes some people anxious

A significant portion of the population carries a variant of a gene called **COMT** — catechol-O-methyltransferase — informally the worry gene. People with this variant process the antioxidant compounds in green tea more slowly.[20] For slow processors, green tea can produce more jitteriness than coffee — the opposite of what you'd expect. People with PTSD are significantly more likely to carry this variant.[19]

The fix is magnesium and vitamin B6 as pyridoxal-5-phosphate. Both nutrients increase COMT enzyme activity.[19] Since adding both to my daily routine — particularly magnesium glycinate at night, consistently — I can drink green tea without the jitters entirely. The self-screening question: does green tea make you feel more wired or anxious rather than calm? If yes, fix the COMT with magnesium and P5P first.

Jasmine — *the herb that works through your nose*

Jasmine is an unusual entry in this chapter because its most documented mechanism isn't something you swallow — it's something you smell. Your olfactory system has a direct neurological pathway to the limbic system, the brain's emotional processing center. Aromatic compounds from jasmine reach the limbic system almost immediately, which is why jasmine can shift mood and anxiety levels faster than anything you take orally.

Research confirms that jasmine aromatherapy enhances feelings of well-being and produces measurable calming effects on the nervous system.[24] A review found that jasmine tea improves mood with both calming and mildly invigorating effects simultaneously.[25] In Ayurvedic medicine, jasmine has been classified for centuries as a cooling herb — one that calms excess heat in the nervous system, soothes inflammation, and brings the body back toward equilibrium.

Organic decaffeinated jasmine tea is widely available and one of my personal evening teas for winding down without feeling flattened. A few drops of jasmine essential oil in a diffuser in the evening is an easy addition to a bedtime routine that costs almost nothing. The ritual of making something beautiful and fragrant at the end of a hard day is doing real physiological work. Jasmine happens to be both.

Jujube — *the fruit you've never heard of that does 71 things*

A friend introduced me to jujube a few years ago, and my first reaction was mild skepticism followed by genuine surprise. Jujube — also called red dates, though unrelated to the dates in the grocery store — is a small, sweet fruit that has been used in traditional Chinese medicine for centuries as a sleep aid, anxiety remedy, and general vitality tonic. It is also, according to a comprehensive review paper, documented to reduce anxiety symptoms through 71 distinct mechanisms.[26]

Seventy-one. I include that number not as hyperbole but because it genuinely reflects how pharmacologically complex this fruit is — multiple alkaloids, flavonoids, saponins, and polysaccharides all working through different pathways simultaneously.

Jujube isn't easy to find in mainstream grocery stores, but it's widely available online and in Asian grocery stores. Dried jujube is the most practical form — soak in water for 10 to 15 minutes, discard the seeds, and use the fruit in teas, soups, or baked goods. The flavor is gently sweet with a slight tartness — simmered into an evening tea with cinnamon and ginger and a little honey, one of the more pleasant ways to support sleep in this entire chapter.

Kava — *the relaxation tea that actually relaxes you*

Kava bars are opening in cities across the United States, and if you've wandered into one wondering what the fuss is about, the answer is simple: kava works. Not in a subtle, give-it-six-weeks way. A review of 11 clinical studies confirms what Pacific Island cultures have known empirically for centuries: kava root meaningfully reduces anxiety symptoms with a strong safety profile.[12] The World Health Organization agrees on the safety question.[49]

Kava's active compounds, called kavalactones, work on GABA receptors in the brain — the same receptors targeted by benzodiazepines, but through a different pathway and without the dependency, cognitive impairment, or withdrawal problems. It's genuinely relaxing without being sedating in a pharmaceutical sense.

- **Drink the tea, skip the supplements.** Only the root is safe — the leaves are toxic, and some supplements have used aerial parts of the plant. Traditional kava root tea uses the root only.
- **This is a stay-home tea.** Kava is genuinely, noticeably relaxing. Do not drink it before driving. It's a wind-down tool, not a midday supplement.
- **The taste is an acquired one.** Earthy, slightly numbing, distinctly unusual. Most commercial kava teas blend it with ginger, cinnamon, and coconut. If your first cup seems strange, give it another try.

Pair it with magnesium glycinate at bedtime and you have two of the most evidence-backed, non-habit-forming relaxation tools available working together.

Lavender — *the original chill pill*

Lavender gets filed under "spa ambiance" by most people, which is a significant underestimation of what it actually does. This is one of the most clinically documented herbs in this entire chapter.

Start with the cortisol finding: in a study of 90 patients preparing for heart surgery — a population under about as much acute stress as it's possible to be under — inhaling lavender essential oil reduced cortisol levels by 70%

compared to the control group.[27] That's not a subtle effect.

A multi-center randomized trial found that Silexan — an oral lavender supplement — reduced anxiety as effectively as lorazepam (a prescription benzodiazepine), without causing sedation, dependency, or withdrawal.[26,27] A second independent study replicated these findings.[28] Replication matters — it's the difference between an interesting result and a reliable one. Lavender clears that bar.

The mechanisms are multiple: linalool reduces inflammatory markers and brain toxic burden;[28] serotonin transporter modulation contributes to antidepressant effects;[27] NMDA receptor blockade protects against cortisol-related nerve toxicity.[28] Lavender also outperformed placebo for menstrual pain in three placebo-controlled trials[29] and shows meaningful benefit for migraine pain.

Lavender is one of the few herbs that works effectively through multiple delivery routes: aromatherapy for immediate acute stress, oral supplementation for sustained anxiety management, and topical for pain. Most people are already using it in one form — closing the gap to therapeutic effect is mostly a matter of dose and intention.

Lemon balm — *the mint's cheerful, citrusy cousin*

If mint is the cool, focused member of the herb family, lemon balm is the one who shows up bright-eyed, smells like sunshine, and somehow manages to be both calming and energizing at the same time. Closely related botanically — same leaf shape, similar growing habits — but where mint goes sharp and cool, lemon balm goes citrusy and warm. It's delicious in salads, excellent with chicken and roasted vegetables, and makes one of the better herbal teas in this entire chapter.

Lemon balm works primarily by raising GABA levels in the body through rosmarinic acid — the same GABA-enhancing polyphenol found in mint, rosemary, thyme, oregano, and sage.[1,2] This explains most of its documented effects: reduced anxiety, improved sleep, relief from heart palpitations, and reduction in nerve pain. A review study confirmed benefits for both anxiety and depression symptoms,[1] and across six separate clinical studies, lemon balm extract consistently produced improvements in mood, memory, alertness, and mental processing alongside the calming effects.[1,2]

Here's what makes lemon balm unusual in the anxiety herb category: it doesn't trade calm for clarity. Most pharmaceutical anxiety treatments produce relaxation at the cost of cognitive sharpness. Lemon balm appears to do both simultaneously — improving brain function while reducing anxiety rather than sedating the problem into submission.[1,2]

Safety profile is as clean as it gets. Long-term use at high doses produced consistent calming effects without notable side effects.[1,2] Grow it in a pot on a windowsill if you have one — it's nearly impossible to kill and perpetually useful.

Licorice root — *the herb that breaks the rules*

Almost everything in this chapter is here because it lowers cortisol. Licorice root is here because sometimes that's the wrong goal.

For people with cortisol resistance or adrenal fatigue — where the problem isn't too much cortisol but a system so depleted it can no longer respond to cortisol properly — licorice root does something none of the other herbs in this chapter do: it raises circulating cortisol levels by slowing the enzyme that breaks cortisol down. For an exhausted adrenal system, that's not a problem. That's the point. Think of it as giving your adrenals a chance to catch their breath.

Beyond cortisol, licorice root has a genuinely broad therapeutic profile: it reduces heartburn, soothes upset stomach, helps with hot flashes, supports respiratory health during coughs and infections, and has early research suggesting benefits for fear, anxiety symptoms, and depression. It also potentiates valerian root — meaning the two taken together work more effectively than either alone, which makes licorice a useful addition to an evening herbal protocol for people who are running on empty rather than running hot.

The safety profile requires more attention here than with most herbs in this chapter. Licorice root is safe short-term, but long-term use can lower potassium levels and raise blood pressure. This is one herb where working with a naturopath or functional medicine practitioner is genuinely worth the extra step. If adrenal fatigue or cortisol resistance sounds like your situation, this one is worth a conversation with a knowledgeable provider.

Magnolia bark — *a margarita without the morning after*

Magnolia bark doesn't get the attention it deserves, possibly because "bark" is not a compelling wellness word and possibly because the supplement industry hasn't figured out how to put it in a celebrity smoothie yet. Both are oversights worth correcting.

The active compound is magnolol, a potent antioxidant that works as a nootropic — protecting nerve tissue, reducing cortisol, and improving the brain's overall resilience to stress.[32] A clinical study found that Relora, a combination of magnolia and phellodendron bark, reduced cortisol, lowered fatigue, improved mood, and increased vigor.[30] A second independent study confirmed the anxiety-reducing effects.[31] Beyond stress, early research suggests benefits for Alzheimer's risk reduction, menopause symptoms, sleep quality, and cancer risk reduction.[33]

Personal account

I tried Relora for the first time on an ordinary afternoon and decided, in my infinite scientific wisdom, that the mall was a perfectly reasonable place to go shortly afterward. Within about an hour I was drifting serenely through department stores with the relaxed, unhurried energy of someone who has had exactly one very good margarita — pleasantly warm, mildly fuzzy around the edges, entirely unbothered by anything, including the aggressive perfume counter staff. None of the alcohol downsides. Just a very calm afternoon of wandering around looking at things I didn't need with surprising contentment.

I relay this story not as a cautionary tale but as genuinely useful information: Relora works, it works noticeably, and your first experience with it should happen at home on a quiet evening. Once you know how you respond to it, it becomes a useful and manageable tool. The couch is a better starting point than the mall.

Medicinal mushrooms — *first line of defense against cortisol*

If someone comes to me drowning in cortisol — exhausted, anxious, barely keeping up — and I had to pick one thing to recommend while we sorted out everything else, it would probably be Lion's Mane. It's that reliable.

Medicinal mushrooms have been used as food and medicine for thousands of years across multiple cultures, and the modern research is catching up to what traditional practitioners observed: these fungi do genuinely interesting things for the nervous system, gut health, and stress response. My two favorites — the ones I return to again and again with clients and in my own routine — are Lion's Mane and Reishi.

Lion's Mane is the one I won't live without. It reduces anxiety, supports nerve growth, and appears to lower cortisol — but the effect most people notice first is a kind of calm clarity that's different from sedation. Not foggy. Not flattened. Just steadier and more capable than before.

Personal account

I had a client a few years ago working three jobs simultaneously — the kind of schedule that would run most people into the ground within a week. She was managing, barely, but the stress was written all over her face and showing up in her labs. We added Lion's Mane supplements to her routine, and within a short period she came back and told me something had shifted. The three jobs were still three jobs — but manageable in a way they hadn't been before. She described feeling like she could think clearly under pressure without the constant background hum of overwhelm. That's Lion's Mane doing what it does. I've heard versions of that story more times than I can count, and I've experienced the same effect myself. It stays in my daily routine permanently.

Reishi works through a somewhat different pathway — primarily improving serotonin metabolism and supporting gut health — which translates to improved mood, reduced depression symptoms, and a calming effect that's more restorative than stimulating.[27] A study in women with fibromyalgia found that Reishi supplementation increased feelings of happiness and reduced depression symptoms.

For quality, look for brands that use the fruiting body rather than mycelium — Real Mushrooms and FreshCap both meet this standard. Lion's Mane shows up fresh in well-stocked grocery stores at certain times of year. Sautéed in butter it has a texture remarkably similar to scallops — which is either a wonderful surprise or a complete non-sequitur depending on what you were expecting from a stress management chapter.

Mint — *the herb your brain already knows*

There's a reason every spa on earth smells like mint. Your limbic system — the brain's emotional processing center — receives aromatic compounds from mint almost directly through the olfactory nerve, bypassing the usual sensory detours and landing straight in the part of the brain that regulates stress, mood, and memory. Walking past a mint plant in the garden and brushing a leaf with your hand can shift your mood before you've had time to think about it.

The clinical research confirms what your nose has always suspected. Peppermint essential oil aromatherapy meaningfully reduced anxiety in patients recovering from heart surgery[34] — a population not known for being easy to calm — and mint has demonstrated consistent improvements in memory and focus across multiple studies.[35] That cognitive benefit is directly relevant to cortisol: a brain running on chronic stress simply cannot focus properly.

Mint also contains apigenin — the GABA-enhancing flavone — which accounts for its simultaneously relaxing and focusing quality. It calms without sedating, which puts it in a fairly exclusive club of herbs that don't make you choose between being relaxed and being useful. For anyone dealing with IBS, mint pulls double duty: peppermint oil is one of the better-studied natural interventions for gut spasms and IBS pain.

Grow it in a pot. Brew it as tea. Crush a leaf when you're stressed and just smell it for a moment. The bar for using mint therapeutically is genuinely as low as it gets, and it works anyway.

Mucuna — *the happy bean that means business*

Mucuna is the odd one out in this chapter — not an herb, not a spice, but a legume that has quietly accumulated one of the more interesting research profiles in the cortisol and mood space. The reason comes down to one compound: L-DOPA, a direct precursor to dopamine. Not a compound that nudges dopamine production in a general direction — an actual precursor that the brain converts directly into dopamine with minimal metabolic steps in between.

Dopamine depletion is one of the most common and least addressed consequences of chronic stress. Cortisol and dopamine have an inverse relationship: when one goes up persistently, the other tends to come down. The exhaustion, the flatness, the loss of motivation that characterizes burnout isn't just tiredness — it's frequently a dopamine problem, and mucuna addresses it at the source.[36]

Beyond dopamine, mucuna balances testosterone levels, reduces cortisol directly, and improves sexual function.[36] Early research also suggests benefit for Parkinson's disease due to its L-DOPA content — a bean that contains a compound used in neurological disease treatment is not a bean you want to dismiss as a wellness trend.

Mucuna needs proper preparation to be consumed safely as a food — supplements are the more reliable route for therapeutic use. Most people notice an energizing, motivated quality from mucuna — a sense of engagement and drive that's distinct from the calm most other entries in this chapter produce. Take it in the daytime, not in the evening. Predictable downside: as a legume, mucuna can cause gas and bloating in sensitive digestive systems. Introduce it gradually.

Passionflower — *the dramatic name is earned*

Passionflower is one of those herbs that looks exactly like it should be medicinal. The flower itself is extraordinary — an elaborate purple and white construction that seems like it was designed by someone who wanted to make absolutely sure you took it seriously. It turns out the appearance is not misleading. Passionflower has been used for centuries for anxiety, insomnia, and irritability, and the modern research supports all three applications.

Personal account

I had a client — a woman juggling a demanding job, two teenagers, and a husband who apparently didn't know where the dishwasher was — who came to me wound so tight she was having trouble sleeping even when she was exhausted. She'd tried melatonin, which helped her fall asleep but didn't help her stay asleep, and she was understandably reluctant to go the prescription route. I suggested passionflower tea as an evening ritual — nothing dramatic, just a cup about an hour before bed. She came back two weeks later visibly different. Calmer. Sleeping longer. Less likely, she reported, to mentally compose strongly-worded emails to her husband at 2am. Passionflower won't reorganize anyone's household labor, but it will take the edge off the part of your nervous system that's still running threat assessments at midnight when you're trying to sleep.

The research backs up what I see clinically. Passionflower reduces stress symptoms when used alongside conventional antidepressant treatment, suggesting it works through complementary rather than competing pathways.[46] It also improves total sleep time — not just sleep onset, but duration — which distinguishes it from herbs that primarily help you fall asleep without extending how long you stay there.[46]

Safety profile is clean for most people. Two exceptions: avoid during pregnancy, and use caution if already taking sedative medications. A warm cup of passionflower tea in the evening is one of the gentler and more pleasant ways to wind down in this entire chapter. It also makes a beautiful tea. Sometimes that matters.

Rhodiola — *the adaptogen for people who are tired of being tired*

Rhodiola has been used as a fatigue remedy across Scandinavia, Russia, and Central Asia for centuries — traditional medicine systems that had little in common culturally but independently arrived at the same root for the same problem. That kind of cross-cultural convergence is worth paying attention to.

What's happening, biochemically, is a fairly elegant set of overlapping actions. Rhodiola increases serotonin activity, promotes a healthy adrenal response, raises GABA levels, and appears to dampen cortisol — the full adaptogenic package, working through several pathways simultaneously rather than targeting a single mechanism.[50] A standardized rhodiola extract reduced symptoms of mild-to-moderate depression better than placebo in a clinical study.[50] For women and men dealing with stress-related hormonal disruption, the cortisol-lowering effect has downstream benefits for essentially every other hormone in the system.

Rhodiola has a distinctive flavor — bitter and slightly sweet, earthy — that pairs reasonably well with ginger or cinnamon if you're making tea. Safety profile is good overall, with two minor caveats: a small number of people experience dizziness or dry mouth,[50] and rhodiola is mildly stimulating, so take it earlier in the day. If you're on SSRIs, check with your provider before adding it — there's a potential interaction worth being aware of.

For anyone whose primary cortisol symptom is the specific exhaustion of having run on stress hormones for too long — the flat, depleted kind rather than the wired kind — rhodiola is one of the more targeted options in this chapter.

Rose — *the medicine hiding in plain sight*

Roses are everywhere. Wedding centerpieces, Valentine's Day obligations, garden borders, perfume counters, and approximately every grandmother's wallpaper pattern since 1974. They are so thoroughly domesticated into decoration that most people have completely forgotten they are also one of the most widely used medicinal plants in human history. This is a significant oversight.

Rose has been used medicinally across Persian, Ayurvedic, Chinese, and European traditional medicine systems for centuries — for mood, for inflammation, for digestive complaints, for grief, for anxiety. It's only in modern "progressive" medicine that rose got demoted from pharmacy to vase.

The clinical research is more substantial than most people expect from a flower. A review of 13 clinical studies found that rose aromatherapy reduces blood pressure, lowers cortisol, decreases adrenaline, reduces anxiety symptoms, and dampens sympathetic nervous system activity — the fight-or-flight response — all from simply being in the presence of the scent.[37] Thirteen studies. That's not a wellness trend. That's a pattern.

Rose tea is one of my personal daily rituals and has been for years — specifically for stress management, and specifically because it works. More research should exist on rose's medicinal properties. It doesn't, for the familiar reason: there's no patent on a rose petal and therefore no financial incentive to fund the trials.[37] What we have is 13 well-designed studies, centuries of consistent traditional use across multiple cultures, and the option to simply try it for ourselves. That's a reasonable enough evidence base for a cup of tea.

Rosemary — *the kitchen herb that's been medicinal all along*

Rosemary is one of those herbs that has been sitting in your spice rack doing considerably more than flavoring roast chicken, and it deserves a proper introduction as the serious medicinal plant it actually is.

Start with the most immediately practical finding: smelling rosemary reduces cortisol levels.[38] Not taking it, not brewing it — smelling it. A study measuring cortisol in saliva found meaningful reductions simply from exposure to rosemary's aromatic compounds, which travel the direct olfactory-to-limbic pathway.[38] The piney, resinous scent that makes rosemary so distinctive in cooking is the same scent doing neurological work on your stress response.

Beyond aromatherapy, rosemary contains rosmarinic acid — the polyphenol shared with mint, lemon balm, thyme, oregano, and sage — which indirectly raises GABA levels and counters the cortisol response.[1,2] It also contains limonene, with its own cortisol-reducing and neuroprotective properties.[22,23] The anti-inflammatory evidence is substantial: carnosic acid and carnosol have demonstrated significant anti-inflammatory effects, reducing inflammatory markers through pathways that overlap with the cortisol-inflammation cycle.[1,2]

Memory and cognitive function are another area where rosemary has accumulated surprisingly strong evidence. Rosemary aromatherapy improved speed and accuracy of mental calculations and improved memory quality in clinical research, effects attributed to the compound 1,8-cineole, which is absorbed through the olfactory system and reaches the brain directly.[35]

Keep a living rosemary plant somewhere you'll walk past and brush the leaves — the scent released by that small contact is doing real work. It has been chronically underused as anything other than a culinary herb. That's worth correcting.

Saffron — *the spice that outperforms its reputation*

Saffron has an image problem. Most people know it as the expensive stuff that turns paella yellow — priced by the gram, used by the pinch, vaguely mysterious in origin. What most people don't know is that it's also one of the most clinically validated natural mood compounds available.

Five clinical trials have demonstrated saffron's antidepressant and anti-anxiety effects at a dose of just 30mg per day.[41] A review of these studies concluded that saffron reduced depression symptoms better than placebo and performed comparably to SSRI medications — without the weight gain, sexual dysfunction, or dependency concerns.[41] The mechanism is distinct from pharmaceutical antidepressants: saffron increases BDNF — brain-derived neurotrophic factor — and nerve growth factor, supporting the actual structural health of the brain rather than just adjusting its chemistry.[41]

Personal account

I use saffron with a significant number of my clients dealing with mood issues, anxiety, and cortisol dysregulation, and the consistency of the results continues to impress me. Clients report feeling more even, less reactive, sleeping better, and handling stress with more resilience. Several have described it as feeling like themselves again rather than feeling medicated. That distinction matters enormously to people who have spent time on SSRIs and didn't like what they found there.

I also take it myself daily, as part of my own mental health and cortisol management routine. Thirty milligrams. Consistent. It's one of the things I genuinely would not want to be without.

At 30mg per day, saffron is also considerably more affordable than its culinary reputation suggests. One absolute contraindication: saffron is not safe during pregnancy and must be avoided entirely in that context.[41]

Sage — *the wise herb that earns its name*

Sage has been associated with wisdom for so long that the association has become a cliché. What gets lost in the metaphor is that the original connection wasn't poetic. It was medicinal. Cultures that used sage regularly observed that it supported memory, clarity, and emotional stability. They called it wise because it made people function better. The modern research is now explaining why.

Personal account

One of my more memorable experiences with sage involved a client — a person with PTSD whose sleep had been fractured for years. Not just difficulty falling asleep, but the kind of sleep disruption that leaves people exhausted and on edge, cycling through the same traumatic material night after night without resolution. We had been working through a comprehensive protocol together, and sage was one of the additions I suggested specifically for its cortisol-reducing and calming properties. He was skeptical — understandably, given that he'd tried a lot of things — but willing to a sage supplement at night.

A few weeks later he came back and told me something had shifted. He was falling asleep more easily, staying asleep longer, and waking up feeling less like he'd spent the night in a fight. Not cured — PTSD doesn't work that way — but measurably better. He'd also started drinking sage tea in the evenings as part of a wind-down ritual. The calming compounds and the ritual of making something warm and quiet before bed working together, in the way that the best herbal approaches tend to.

The research supports what I observed with him. Inhaling sage essential oil reduces cortisol levels and produces antidepressant effects — documented in menopausal women, a population dealing with significant hormonal stress, but the cortisol-reducing mechanism is not population-specific.[39]

The memory benefits are well-documented for a culinary herb. A six-week clinical trial in healthy adults found that sage improved both short- and long-term memory, with multiple additional studies confirming the finding extends to people with dementia as well.[40] The mechanism: sage slows the breakdown of acetylcholine, a neurotransmitter critical for memory consolidation — the same mechanism targeted by some Alzheimer's medications, without the side effect profile.

Dosing note: common sage contains thujone, which is safe in normal amounts but warrants attention at high doses long-term. Stay at or under the equivalent of three to six cups of sage tea daily, or under 600mg of oral supplements.[39] Spanish sage contains no thujone and can be used without this consideration.

Skullcap — *the earthy nightcap that earns its name*

Skullcap is a mint family herb that does several useful things simultaneously, characteristic of the flavonoid-rich herbs throughout this chapter. Its primary antioxidants are flavonoids — including apigenin — that reduce inflammation, dampen cortisol release from the adrenal glands directly,[42] and bind GABA receptors to produce genuine anti-anxiety effects.[43] These same flavonoids appear to reduce histamine release, making skullcap quietly useful for people whose stress comes packaged with allergies or immune reactivity.

The sleep research is solid. A clinical study found that 400mg daily improved sleep quality, total sleep time, and time to fall asleep in people with insomnia.[51] A separate trial found that skullcap significantly improved mood compared to placebo.[44] Better sleep and better mood through overlapping mechanisms — a useful option for people whose cortisol symptoms show up primarily at night.

Two practical notes: start at the lowest effective dose and increase only if needed — more is genuinely not better here.[42] And because skullcap can interact with certain prescription medications, this is one worth running by your provider before starting, particularly if you're on anything for anxiety, sleep, or liver conditions.[44]

Tulsi (holy basil) — *the herb I would take to a desert island*

If I could only keep one herbal tea in my life, it would be tulsi. I am not being dramatic. This herb has been my daily stress management ritual for years, and it earns its place every single day. Combined with rose — which it pairs with beautifully, both in flavor and in mechanism — it is the most reliably calming cup I know.

Tulsi, also called holy basil, is related to the sweet basil you put on pizza, but it has been doing considerably more interesting work in Ayurvedic medicine for several thousand years. A review of 24 clinical studies confirmed what traditional practitioners observed empirically: tulsi manages stress, reduces blood pressure, improves immune function, and reduces fatigue — with no major side effects across the entire body of research.[45] Twenty-four studies. No major side effects. For an herb that does that many things, that's a remarkable safety profile.

The mechanism involves the same adaptogenic pathways that run through several herbs in this chapter — tulsi helps the body regulate its cortisol response rather than simply suppressing it, which means it works with your stress system rather than against it. It's calming without being sedating, energizing without being stimulating, and manages to do both at the same time in a way that most herbs — and essentially all pharmaceuticals — can't quite pull off.

Making tulsi tea is as simple as it gets: boiling water, tulsi tea bags or loose leaf, five minutes of steeping, done. Add a rose tea bag and a small drizzle of honey if you want something that tastes like it was made by someone who genuinely cares about you. One caution: tulsi carries a theoretical risk of increased bleeding when taken alongside blood thinners.[45] If you're on anticoagulant medication, skip this one and talk to your provider about alternatives. For everyone else — go make a cup right now. Seriously.

Valerian root — *the dependable sleep herb with daytime uses too*

Valerian root is the herb most people have heard of for sleep, and for good reason. It's one of the most well-studied natural sleep aids available, with multiple clinical trials confirming benefits for sleep onset, sleep quality, and total sleep time.[47]

The mechanism is primarily GABA enhancement — valerian's active compounds bind to GABA receptors in the brain in a way that promotes relaxation without the dependency, rebound insomnia, or morning grogginess associated with pharmaceutical sedatives. It works best at doses between 120–400mg taken 30 to 60 minutes before bed. Some people experience mild next-day drowsiness when starting — begin at the lower end of the dose range and adjust.

Valerian's lesser-known application is daytime anxiety management in people with very high cortisol — the kind of chronic, unrelenting stress response that contributes to insomnia in the first place. One clinical review found meaningful reductions in anxiety symptoms with regular valerian use.[48] For people in grief or dealing with significant acute stress, I have found valerian to be one of the more reliable tools for taking the edge off the nervous system during the day while also supporting sleep at night. The smell is notably earthy — some people find it off putting, and that's normal. It doesn't indicate a quality problem.

Licorice root potentiates valerian, as mentioned in the licorice entry — the two taken together work more effectively than either alone, a useful combination for people dealing with adrenal fatigue alongside sleep issues.

Violets — *yes, you can eat them*

I am a registered dietitian recommending that you eat flowers. We have arrived.

Violets — the common purple ones that appear in yards and gardens in spring — are edible, antioxidant-rich, anti-inflammatory, and have a long traditional history as a calming herb for anxiety and nervous conditions. The flavonoids in violet petals include rutin and quercetin, compounds with documented anti-inflammatory and antioxidant activity.

The research on violets as a cortisol-specific herb is thin — limited funding for studying flowers that everyone already has access to for free — but the anecdotal and traditional evidence for their calming properties is consistent across cultures and centuries. The anti-inflammatory activity is well-documented for the compound class, even if violet-specific trials are sparse.

The practical application couldn't be simpler. Add fresh violet petals to salads for a burst of color and mild floral flavor. Brew them as a simple tea. Candy them with egg white and sugar for a beautiful edible garnish. Forage them from your own lawn or garden if it's unsprayed — they're genuinely easy to identify and genuinely impossible to overdose on.

The most underused cortisol tool in this entire book is probably growing in your backyard right now, for free.

Herb and spice reference tables

The following two tables consolidate all herb information from this chapter. **Table 1** covers herbs, key benefits, dose guidance, and recommended form. **Table 2** covers recommended brands or sources and key cautions. The brand recommendations reflect quality considerations and personal or clinical experience, not commercial relationships.

Chapter 7 herb and spice table — Table 1

Herbs, key cortisol benefits, dose guidance, and recommended form

Herb / Spice	Key cortisol benefits	Dose	Form
Ashwagandha	Reduces cortisol up to 30%; reduces anxiety; improves sleep and thyroid function	300-600 mg daily	Capsule, powder, tincture
Black cumin seed	Reduces cortisol, stress, and anxiety; increases melatonin; GABA-enhancing	200 mg oil daily	Capsule, oil
Cannabis / CBD	Reduces stress, anxiety, PTSD symptoms; improves sleep	5-27 mg CBD daily	Full-spectrum oil, tincture
Cardamom	Reduces cortisol, blood pressure, and inflammatory markers	~1 tsp (3,000 mg) daily	Spice, supplement
Celery	GABA-enhancing; nootropic; reduces cortisol indirectly; anti-inflammatory	1 dropperful tincture daily	Tincture, food, seeds
Chamomile	Reduces anxiety and depression; improves sleep; immediate cortisol effect	3 cups tea daily or 500 mg	Tea, capsule
Feverfew	GABA-enhancing; analgesic; reduces migraines; calming	Tea or 100-300 mg supplement	Tea, capsule, tincture
Ginseng (Panax)	Reduces cortisol; improves mood, focus, testosterone; GABA/serotonin enhancing	100-600 mg AM	Capsule, tea, tincture
Green tea	Reduces anxiety; improves memory; L-theanine balances caffeine stimulation	3-4 cups organic matcha daily	Tea (organic matcha best)
Jasmine	Reduces cortisol, blood pressure, adrenaline; improves mood	Tea or essential oil diffusion	Tea, essential oil, tincture
Jujube	71 documented mechanisms for anxiety reduction; improves sleep and vitality	Soaked dried fruit in tea or food	Dried fruit, tea, supplement
Kava	Reduces anxiety via GABA/kavalactones; promotes relaxation and sleep	Traditional root tea	Root tea only (not supplements)
Lavender	Reduces cortisol 70% (aromatherapy); equals lorazepam for anxiety without dependency	80 mg Silexan or diffuse	Essential oil, supplement, tea
Lemon balm	Reduces anxiety, insomnia, palpitations; improves memory and mood; GABA-enhancing	300-1,000 mg daily	Supplement, tea, fresh herb
Licorice root	Raises cortisol for adrenal fatigue/resistance; reduces heartburn; potentiates valerian	Low dose short-term only	Tea, tincture, supplement
Magnolia bark	Reduces cortisol; improves sleep, mood, menopause; neuroprotective	250 mg Relora	Supplement (Relora)
Medicinal mushrooms	Lion's Mane: reduces anxiety, cortisol, nerve growth; Reishi: improves mood, serotonin	1,000-2,000 mg daily	Supplement, tea, fresh (Lion's Mane)
Mint	GABA-enhancing via apigenin; reduces anxiety; improves memory and focus; IBS relief	Tea, food, aromatherapy freely	Tea, essential oil, fresh herb
Mucuna	Direct dopamine precursor; reduces cortisol; balances testosterone; improves mood	Start low; supplement form	Capsule (not raw bean)
Passionflower	Reduces stress and anxiety; improves sleep duration; GABA-modulating	Tea before bed or supplement	Tea, capsule, tincture
Rhodiola	Reduces cortisol; improves fatigue, mood, depression; GABA/serotonin enhancing	340-680 mg AM	Capsule, tea, tincture
Rose	Reduces cortisol, blood pressure, adrenaline; reduces anxiety and sympathetic nerve activity	Tea daily; essential oil diffusion	Tea, essential oil, tincture
Rosemary	Reduces cortisol (aromatherapy); GABA-enhancing via rosmarinic acid; improves memory	Cook fresh, supplement or diffuse	Fresh herb, essential oil, supplement
Saffron	Reduces depression and anxiety; equals SSRIs; increases BDNF and nerve growth factor	30 mg daily	Capsule, spice
Sage	Reduces cortisol; antidepressant; improves memory and sleep; acetylcholinesterase inhibitor	3-6 cups tea or under 600 mg	Tea, essential oil, capsule
Skullcap	Reduces cortisol from adrenal glands; GABA-binding; improves sleep quality and mood	400 mg daily	Capsule, tea, tincture
Tulsi (holy basil)	Reduces stress, blood pressure, fatigue; improves immunity; calming without sedating	Tea or 250 mg supplement	Tea, capsule, tincture
Valerian root	Reduces anxiety and insomnia; GABA-enhancing; reduces cortisol markers	120-400 mg or tea at night	Tea, capsule, tincture
Violets	Antioxidant-rich; anti-inflammatory; anecdotally calming; edible flowers	Eat petals in food or tea freely	Edible flower, tea

CHAPTER 7

Chapter 7 herb and spice table — Table 2

Recommended brands or sources and key cautions

Herb / Spice	Recommended brands / sources	Cautions
Ashwagandha	KSM-66 or Sensoril standardized extracts; many quality brands	Avoid in pregnancy. Can lower thyroid medication effectiveness.
Black cumin seed	Now brand black seed oil (consistent quality per personal experience)	No major side effects at research doses.
Cannabis / CBD	Full-spectrum oil from reputable dispensary; Charlotte's Web, Medterra	Not for driving. Variable legal status. Strain variation significant.
Cardamom	Organic green cardamom from spice stores	Very safe. Limit if on anticoagulants at very high doses.
Celery	Celery seed tincture (author uses daily); celery seed extract capsules	Very safe. Caution in severe kidney disease (potassium).
Chamomile	Alvita, Traditional Medicinals, or any organic loose chamomile	Avoid if sensitive to daisy/ragweed family. Safe in pregnancy.
Feverfew	MigreLief, Nature's Answer; many quality capsule brands	Don't chew raw leaves. Avoid if sensitive to daisy family.
Ginseng (Panax)	Look for Panax ginseng specifically on label; Jarrow, Now brands	Stimulating — take AM only. American ginseng not equivalent. Indian ginseng = ashwagandha.
Green tea	Organic matcha; Ippodo, Aiya brands for quality	COMT gene variant may cause jitteriness — fix with magnesium + P5P first.
Jasmine	Organic decaffeinated jasmine tea; NOW jasmine essential oil	Very safe. Avoid high-dose supplements in pregnancy.
Jujube	Dried jujube from Asian grocery or online; health food stores	Very safe. Soak and discard seeds for food use.
Kava	Traditional root tea only. Kona Kava Farm; Fiji Kava	Avoid supplements (leaf contamination risk). Don't drive after use. Avoid in pregnancy.
Lavender	Silexan supplement (80 mg); NOW or Plant Therapy essential oils	Very safe. Oral supplements more concentrated than tea.
Lemon balm	Gaia Herbs, Herb Pharm, Traditional Medicinals	Very safe long-term. Pairs well with chamomile or tulsi.
Licorice root	Traditional Medicinals tea; Herb Pharm tincture	Short-term use only. Monitor blood pressure and potassium. Work with provider.
Magnolia bark	Relora by Source Naturals (clinically tested combination)	Start at home. Mildly sedating. Very safe.
Medicinal mushrooms	Real Mushrooms or FreshCap (fruiting body, not mycelium)	Very safe. Saute fresh Lion's Mane in butter for culinary use.
Mint	Fresh or dried; any organic brand	Very safe. Peppermint oil capsules for IBS (enteric coated).
Mucuna	NOW Sports mucuna pruriens; Banyan Botanicals	Start low. Can be stimulating. May cause gas in sensitive people.
Passionflower	Herb Pharm, Gaia Herbs; Traditional Medicinals tea	Avoid in pregnancy. Caution with sedative medications.
Rhodiola	Rhodiola rosea standardized to 3% rosavins; Gaia Herbs, Herb Pharm	Take AM. May interact with SSRIs. Dizziness or dry mouth in some.
Rose	Organic rose petal tea; Rose essential oil (any quality brand)	Very safe. No patent on a rose petal — just try it.
Rosemary	Fresh from garden or store; rosemary essential oil for diffusion	Very safe in food and aromatherapy quantities.
Saffron	Pharmavite Safr'Inside or Life Extension saffron (30 mg standardized)	Avoid in pregnancy (absolute contraindication). Very safe otherwise.
Sage	Common sage tea; Spanish sage supplement (no thujone)	Limit common sage to 600 mg/day long-term (thujone). Spanish sage has no limit.
Skullcap	Herb Pharm, Gaia Herbs skullcap tincture	Check with provider if on prescription medications. Rare liver interaction.
Tulsi (holy basil)	Organic India Tulsi tea (author's daily tea); capsules widely available	Theoretical bleeding risk with anticoagulants. Very safe otherwise.
Valerian root	Traditional Medicinals, Gaia Herbs; often combined with lemon balm	Earthy smell (normal). Some feel next-day grogginess — start low.
Violets	Forage from unsprayed areas or grow in garden	Very safe. Eat freely. Consult if foraging — make sure of identification.

References

1 Rosmarinic acid and GABA. Phytomedicine. 2010. https://pubmed.ncbi.nlm.nih.gov/20739071/

2 Rosmarinic acid and anxiety. Phytother Res. 2019. https://pubmed.ncbi.nlm.nih.gov/31140674/

3 Ashwagandha and cortisol. Medicine (Baltimore). 2019. https://pubmed.ncbi.nlm.nih.gov/31517876/

4 Black cumin seed, cortisol, and melatonin. Phytother Res. 2021. https://pubmed.ncbi.nlm.nih.gov/34491595/

5 CBD and stress. Neurotherapeutics. 2015. https://pmc.ncbi.nlm.nih.gov/articles/PMC4604171/

6 CBD dose-response. Front Psychiatry. 2021. https://pmc.ncbi.nlm.nih.gov/articles/PMC7861010/

7 Cannabis and PTSD. J Psychoactive Drugs. 2014. https://pubmed.ncbi.nlm.nih.gov/25052497/

8 Cannabis and PTSD outcomes. J Clin Psychol. 2019. https://pubmed.ncbi.nlm.nih.gov/28852907/

9 Cannabis and sleep. Medicines (Basel). 2018. https://pmc.ncbi.nlm.nih.gov/articles/PMC6326553/

10 Cardamom meta-analysis and cortisol. Phytother Res. 2023. https://pubmed.ncbi.nlm.nih.gov/36597913/

11 Chamomile and anxiety/depression. Phytomedicine. 2017. https://pubmed.ncbi.nlm.nih.gov/28483761/

12 Kava and anxiety. Cochrane Database Syst Rev. 2003. https://pubmed.ncbi.nlm.nih.gov/12804413/

13 Feverfew and stress/inflammation. Molecules. 2021. https://pmc.ncbi.nlm.nih.gov/articles/PMC8233473/

14 Feverfew and migraines. Cochrane Database Syst Rev. 2004. https://pubmed.ncbi.nlm.nih.gov/15495046/

18 Green tea and anxiety. Phytomedicine. 2017. https://pubmed.ncbi.nlm.nih.gov/27825024/

19 COMT gene and PTSD. J Psychiatr Res. 2018. https://pubmed.ncbi.nl

m.nih.gov/30098547/

20 COMT and catechin processing. Am J Clin Nutr. 2010. https://pubmed.ncbi.nlm.nih.gov/20016016/

21 Ginseng, testosterone, and cortisol. J Ginseng Res. 2013. https://pmc.ncbi.nlm.nih.gov/articles/PMC3659620/

22 Ginseng and cognitive function. Nutrients. 2022. https://pubmed.ncbi.nlm.nih.gov/35276829/

23 Ginseng GABA and serotonin. J Ethnopharmacol. 2021. https://pubmed.ncbi.nlm.nih.gov/32861833/

24 Jasmine aromatherapy and well-being. Eur Neuropsychopharmacol. 2010. https://pubmed.ncbi.nlm.nih.gov/20569508/

25 Jasmine tea and mood. J Biol Chem. 2010. https://pubmed.ncbi.nlm.nih.gov/20565767/

26 Jujube and anxiety mechanisms. J Ethnopharmacol. 2019. https://pubmed.ncbi.nlm.nih.gov/30528663/

27 Lavender and cortisol. Complement Ther Med. 2015. https://pubmed.ncbi.nlm.nih.gov/27563324/

28 Silexan versus lorazepam. Phytomedicine. 2010. https://pubmed.ncbi.nlm.nih.gov/19962288/

29 Lavender and menstrual pain. Int J Gynaecol Obstet. 2015. https://pubmed.ncbi.nlm.nih.gov/25571308/

30 Relora and cortisol. J Int Soc Sports Nutr. 2008. https://pubmed.ncbi.nlm.nih.gov/18950526/

31 Relora and anxiety. Altern Ther Health Med. 2001. https://pubmed.ncbi.nlm.nih.gov/11347281/

32 Magnolol neuroprotection. Front Pharmacol. 2019. https://pmc.ncbi.nlm.nih.gov/articles/PMC6763605/

33 Magnolia and Alzheimer's. Curr Alzheimer Res. 2020. https://pubmed.ncbi.nlm.nih.gov/32175839/

34 Peppermint aromatherapy post-cardiac surgery. Complement Ther Med. 2020. https://pubmed.ncbi.nlm.nih.gov/33007223/

35 Mint and memory/cognitive function. Int J Neurosci. 2008. https://pubmed.ncbi.nlm.nih.gov/18444144/

36 Mucuna and cortisol. Fertil Steril. 2008. https://pubmed.ncbi.nlm.nih.gov/18068175/

37 Rose aromatherapy review. Complement Ther Clin Pract. 2019. https://pubmed.ncbi.nlm.nih.gov/31331614/

38 Rosemary aromatherapy and cortisol. Psychiatry Res. 2007. https://pubmed.ncbi.nlm.nih.gov/17291598/

39 Sage and cortisol. Complement Ther Med. 2016. https://pubmed.ncbi.nlm.nih.gov/26471072/

40 Sage and memory. Pharmacol Biochem Behav. 2003. https://pubmed.ncbi.nlm.nih.gov/12867266/

41 Saffron and depression meta-analysis. J Integr Med. 2019. https://pubmed.ncbi.nlm.nih.gov/31405673/

42 Apigenin and GABA/cortisol. Phytomedicine. 2017. https://pubmed.ncbi.nlm.nih.gov/28236605/

43 Skullcap GABA binding. Altern Ther Health Med. 2003. https://pubmed.ncbi.nlm.nih.gov/12929243/

44 Skullcap and mood. Altern Ther Health Med. 2014. https://pubmed.ncbi.nlm.nih.gov/24614320/

45 Tulsi review: 24 clinical studies. J Ayurveda Integr Med. 2017. https://pmc.ncbi.nlm.nih.gov/articles/PMC5376420/

46 Passionflower and sleep/anxiety. J Clin Pharm Ther. 2011. https://pubmed.ncbi.nlm.nih.gov/21294203/

47 Valerian and sleep. Am J Med. 2006. https://pubmed.ncbi.nlm.nih.gov/16569589/

48 Valerian and anxiety. Phytother Res. 2018. https://pubmed.ncbi.nlm.nih.gov/29086589/

49 WHO report on kava safety. World Health Organization. 2007. https://www.who.int/publications/i/item/9789241596862

50 Rhodiola and adaptogens. Front Pharmacol. 2022. https://pmc.ncbi.nlm.nih.gov/articles/PMC9228580/

51 Skullcap and insomnia. Altern Ther Health Med. 2014. https://pubmed.ncbi.nlm.nih.gov/24855047/

8

Chapter 8

CHAPTER 8

WHEN IN DOUBT, FIX YOUR GUT

If there's one chapter in this book where I want you to lean in and read every word, it's this one.

Not because the gut is the most dramatic system in the body — it's not, it's largely invisible until something goes wrong. But because the relationship between gut health and cortisol is both more powerful and more bidirectional than most people realize, and because in my 26 years of clinical practice, addressing the gut has consistently been the most reliable route to meaningful, lasting cortisol improvement. Not the most glamorous route. The most reliable one.

This chapter covers the research on probiotics and cortisol, the hidden problem of bacterial overgrowth, the role of food sensitivities in driving chronic inflammation, what the MRT test actually tells us, and how to rebuild a gut that's been damaged by stress, medications, or both. I'll also cover the clinical picture I see in practice — what gut recovery actually looks like over time — and the hormone DHEA, which is one of the more underused tools in the whole cortisol conversation.

The gut-cortisol loop

Let's revisit the dialogue introduced in Chapter 1, because it bears repeating here in its full version:

Your body's own words

Cortisol: "Hi, I'm cortisol. I'm supposed to be neutralized here, in the gut."

Gut: "Nope, can't do it — you ate too much sugar and you don't have enough probiotics and nutrients to neutralize that cortisol."

Cortisol: "Fine, we'll go back into the bloodstream and be 'extra.' We'll see how you like that, body!"

Body: "Why am I gaining weight, having mood swings, bloating, acne, and insomnia?"

Gut: "Get me back on track and then we can help fix that cortisol, which is causing most of your problems."

Cortisol: "Fine, I'll just raise blood sugar then."

Gut: "I literally cannot with you right now."

That dialogue is not a metaphor. It is a simplified but mechanistically accurate description of how cortisol and the gut interact when things have gone sideways. Your gut genuinely is where cortisol gets metabolized and neutralized. When the gut is compromised — by stress, by poor diet, by medications, by dysbiosis — cortisol recirculates rather than being cleared. The elevated cortisol then further damages the gut. The gut damage worsens cortisol clearance. Repeat until someone finally addresses the underlying problem.

That underlying problem is what this chapter is about.

KEY INSIGHT

The gut is not just a passive recipient of the stress response. It is an active participant in regulating it. When your gut is healthy, it helps clear cortisol. When it isn't, cortisol accumulates. Fixing the gut is not adjacent to fixing your cortisol — it is central to it.

The hidden problem: when the wrong bacteria win

Most conversations about gut health and cortisol focus on what's missing — the beneficial bacteria that aren't there, the probiotics that haven't been added yet. That's an important part of the picture. But there's a second part that gets considerably less attention: the bacteria that are there but shouldn't be, or that are there in excessive amounts.

Bacterial overgrowth is more common than most people realize and considerably more consequential for the cortisol response than the conventional medical conversation acknowledges. When the wrong bacteria colonize the gut, they drive ongoing immune activation, inflammatory signaling, and the kind of low-grade systemic stress that keeps cortisol elevated regardless of what else you're doing.

Personal account

I've dealt with this personally. For a period of time, I was experiencing symptoms I couldn't quite account for — lingering fatigue, digestive irregularity, mood that wasn't responding the way it should have to my supplement regimen. I eventually tracked it down to a Streptococcus overgrowth in my gut.

The solution was berberine — a plant compound with potent antimicrobial and gut-balancing properties that I've come to regard as one of the most underused tools in functional gut medicine. I took berberine at therapeutic doses for a defined protocol period, combined with a quality probiotic to restore beneficial bacteria after clearing the overgrowth, and the difference was significant. The symptoms resolved. The mood and energy that had been slightly off-baseline returned to where they should be.

I've since used berberine with numerous clients dealing with similar presentations — particularly those whose cortisol symptoms aren't responding to the nutritional interventions that usually work. In many cases, bacterial overgrowth is the missing piece. Fix the gut ecology, and the cortisol picture improves.

Berberine: the gut-balancing compound worth knowing

Berberine is a natural alkaloid found in several plants including barberry, goldenseal, and Oregon grape. It has been used in traditional Chinese and Ayurvedic medicine for thousands of years, primarily for digestive complaints and infections, and the modern research is beginning to explain why with considerable precision.

Berberine has documented antimicrobial activity against a range of pathogenic bacteria while showing selectivity that spares or supports beneficial Lactobacillus and Bifidobacterium species.[15] This selectivity is what makes it particularly useful for overgrowth situations — it doesn't carpet-bomb the microbiome the way antibiotics tend to. It reduces the overgrowth while protecting the beneficial populations you want to preserve.

Beyond its antimicrobial properties, berberine reduces gut inflammation, improves the integrity of the gut lining, and has demonstrated meaningful effects on blood sugar regulation and insulin sensitivity.[16] For people whose cortisol dysregulation has contributed to insulin resistance — which is a significant portion of chronically stressed people — berberine addresses both the gut ecology and the metabolic downstream effects simultaneously.

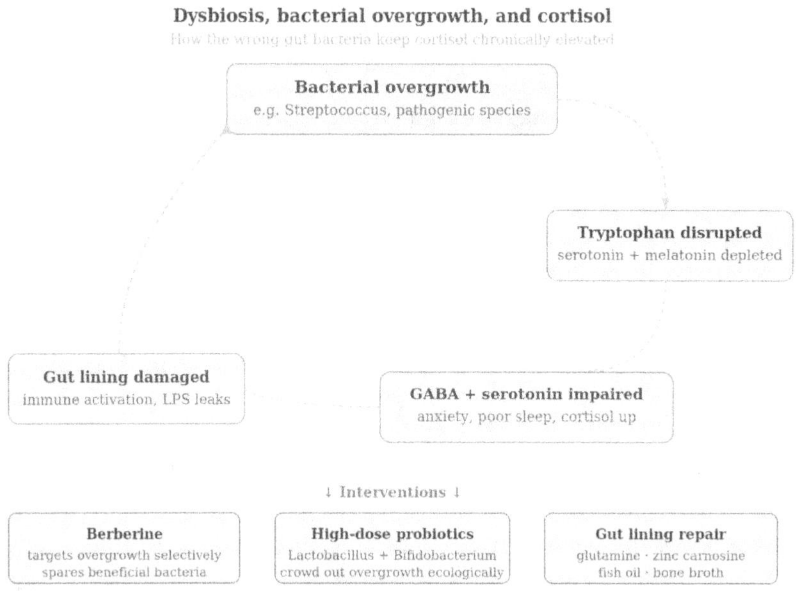

Diagram: Bacterial overgrowth and the cortisol cycle — showing: dysbiotic bacteria → immune activation → inflammatory signaling → cortisol elevation → gut lining damage → further dysbiosis → loop continues. Berberine shown as intervention breaking the overgrowth link; probiotic shown as restoration after clearance.

Food sensitivities — the leaky gut accelerant nobody talks about

If you've been doing everything right — probiotics, anti-inflammatory diet, quality supplements, stress management — and your symptoms still aren't fully resolving, food sensitivities are one of the first places I look. They are one of the most common hidden drivers of persistent gut inflammation and cortisol dysregulation, and they are almost entirely ignored by conventional medicine.

The reason they get ignored is partly methodological. Food sensitivities are not the same as food allergies. An allergic reaction is immediate and unmistakable — your throat closes, your skin breaks out, you know within minutes. A sensitivity reaction is delayed, diffuse, and highly individual. It might show up as bloating four hours after eating. It might show up as a headache the next morning. It might show up as mood instability or joint pain or a cortisol spike that has no obvious trigger. The connection between the food and the symptom is almost impossible to identify without systematic testing because the timing and the symptom profile are both so variable.

When you eat a food you're sensitive to, your immune system responds to it as a threat. This triggers the release of inflammatory mediators — chemicals that cause the full spectrum of inflammatory symptoms — and simultaneously activates your stress response. Cortisol rises. For people with multiple sensitivities eating reactive foods multiple times a day, this produces a state of chronic low-grade immune activation that looks exactly like — and contributes directly to — chronic cortisol dysregulation.

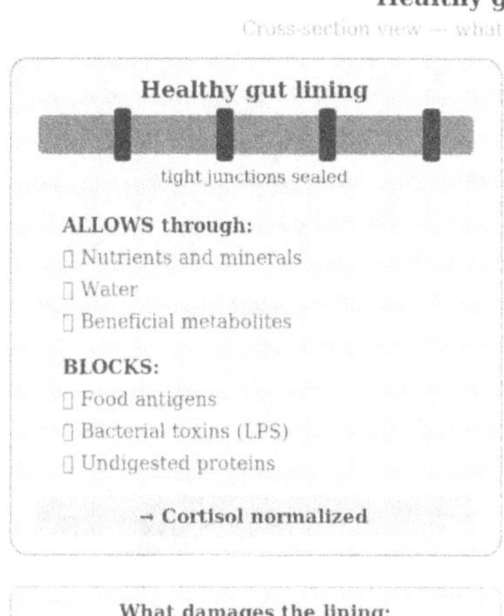
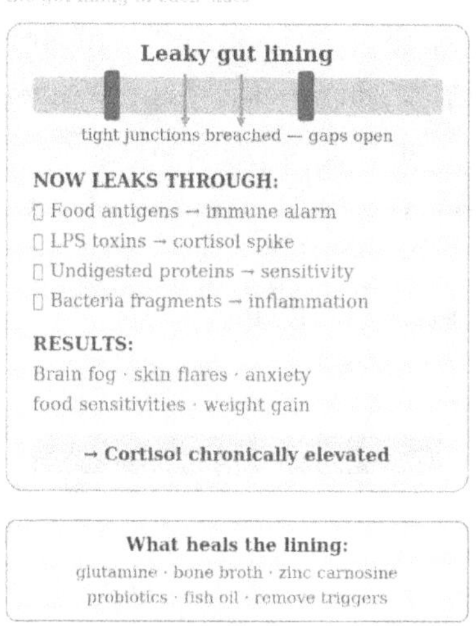

Testing that actually finds the problem: the MRT

The **Mediator Release Test** — MRT — is the most clinically useful food sensitivity test I've worked with in 26 years of practice. It measures the actual release of inflammatory mediators from white blood cells in response to 176 foods and food chemicals — not just the presence of antibodies, which is what most IgG tests measure and why most IgG tests produce results that are simultaneously expensive and unreliable.

The distinction matters practically. IgG antibodies indicate exposure, not reaction. You can have IgG antibodies to dozens of foods and have no sensitivity to any of them. The MRT measures what actually happens when your immune cells encounter each food — whether they release the inflammatory mediators that drive symptoms. That's a fundamentally different question, and it produces results that are actionable in a way that IgG testing frequently isn't.

MRT vs. IgG food sensitivity testing

MRT measures actual inflammatory mediator release from white blood cells — 176 foods and chemicals tested, high sensitivity and specificity, guides the LEAP anti-inflammatory protocol.

IgG testing measures antibody exposure only — indicates what you've encountered, not what you're reacting to. Frequently flags foods that don't cause symptoms and misses ones that do.

For more information: thehealthyrd.com/how-mrt-testing-transformed-my-health-from-the-inside-out

How dysbiosis and food sensitivities compound each other

Here's where the picture gets more complex and more important. Dysbiosis — imbalanced gut bacteria — contributes directly to food sensitivities by compromising gut lining integrity. When the gut lining is damaged or permeable, food antigens cross into the bloodstream that wouldn't normally be there. The immune system encounters them, mounts a response, and a sensitivity is established.

The food sensitivity then drives ongoing gut inflammation that further damages the gut lining. The further damaged gut lining allows more antigens through. More sensitivities develop. The dysbiosis worsens because the inflammation creates a less hospitable environment for beneficial bacteria. The cortisol that rises in response to all this inflammation further suppresses immune regulation and compromises the gut lining.

This is why the comprehensive approach matters. Treating the dysbiosis without addressing the food sensitivities leaves the immune activation continuing. Treating the food sensitivities without addressing the dysbiosis means the gut lining damage that enabled them continues. Both need to be addressed, ideally in sequence: reduce the inflammatory triggers first, then work to restore the microbiome in a gut environment that's no longer actively attacking it.

What I see in practice: gut recovery and cortisol

Let me tell you what gut recovery actually looks like in clinical practice, because the research summaries in this chapter are important but they don't fully capture what it's like to watch someone's health genuinely shift.

The pattern I see most often goes something like this: a client comes in with a constellation of symptoms that has been attributed to different causes by different practitioners — anxiety here, IBS there, weight that won't respond to diet changes, skin that flares for no apparent reason, sleep that's never quite right. Each symptom has been addressed individually and partially, with moderate success at best.

When we address the gut systematically — identifying and removing reactive foods, addressing any overgrowth, restoring the microbiome with targeted probiotics, healing the gut lining with glutamine and anti-inflammatory nutrients — the symptoms often improve across the board, and not gradually. The improvements come faster than most clients expect, and they come together. The anxiety that was being treated separately gets better when the gut does. The skin clears when the gut inflammation reduces. The weight that wasn't moving starts to move. Sleep improves.

This doesn't happen because the gut is a magic system. It happens because the gut was the common upstream cause of most of the downstream symptoms, and addressing the root changes the picture.

Personal account

One of my more striking clinical experiences in the past few years involved a client who came to me after years of treatment for gut pain, anxiety, and depression that had never fully resolved. She had tried multiple medications, several therapists, dietary changes. She was functional but chronically not herself — the flat, depleted, in pain, sick version of herself rather than the engaged, energetic one.

Her gut history was significant: a period of heavy antibiotic use several years earlier, followed by persistent digestive issues that had been managed with proton pump inhibitors. The combination had left her microbiome substantially disrupted, which had never been specifically addressed. Her doctor told her to go home and relax-it was all in her head.

We worked on her gut over several months. Removed the PPI gradually with provider support. Addressed the dysbiosis. Ran an MRT and identified several reactive foods she removed from her diet while adding in nourishing, calming foods. Added a quality probiotic and a gut healing protocol including glutamine. Her mood began to shift within one week of the dietary changes — more noticeably than it had on any medication she'd tried. By one week she described feeling like she had returned to herself after a long absence. Her cortisol markers improved correspondingly and she had a big smile on her face instead of distress.

Antibiotics and gut restoration

Antibiotics save lives. I want to be clear about that before saying anything else, because the nuanced conversation about antibiotic overuse is sometimes heard as anti-antibiotic, and it's not. When antibiotics are genuinely necessary — for serious bacterial infection, for conditions that won't resolve without them — they should absolutely be used.

The problem is that "genuinely necessary" has expanded considerably over the decades. Antibiotics are routinely prescribed for viral infections they cannot touch, for minor bacterial infections that would resolve without intervention, and often prophylactically in ways that accumulate over a lifetime. The microbiome consequences of this accumulation are real and clinically significant.

A course of broad-spectrum antibiotics can reduce gut bacterial diversity by up to 30% — and diversity is the single most important predictor of a healthy microbiome. Some of that diversity returns naturally over weeks to months. Some of it, depending on the antibiotic and the individual, doesn't return without active intervention.[17]

Active intervention means probiotics — started during the antibiotic course (at a different time of day from the antibiotic dose) and continued for at least four to eight weeks after. It means prebiotic fibers to feed the recovering populations. It means fermented foods where the gut can tolerate them. And it means patience, because microbiome recovery after significant disruption takes months, not weeks.

For people whose stress symptoms worsened noticeably after a course of antibiotics — and this is a pattern I see frequently in practice — the antibiotic disruption may have been the precipitating event as research shows. The microbiome disruption that followed affected the gut-brain axis, altered the cortisol clearance that happens in a healthy gut, and produced the anxiety, mood changes, and stress reactivity that followed. Restoring the microbiome doesn't always fully reverse this — but it frequently improves it significantly, and it's almost always the right first step.

Probiotics reduce anxiety: the clinical research

I want to spend some time on the probiotic research specifically, because it's more substantial than most people realize and because the quality of the evidence matters for making confident clinical recommendations.

The research isn't perfect — no research body ever is, and probiotic research has particular challenges around strain specificity, dose standardization, and outcome measurement. But what exists is coherent and directionally consistent in a way that I find genuinely persuasive.

The research case: anxiety

A systematic review and meta-analysis covering both animal and human studies found that probiotic supplementation significantly reduced anxiety-like behaviors and markers.[1] Multiple mechanisms were proposed, including modulation of the HPA axis — the cortisol-producing stress response system — and direct effects on neurotransmitter production via the gut-brain axis.

A separate clinical trial in healthy volunteers found that a multi-strain probiotic reduced psychological distress and improved cognitive reactivity to sad mood,[2] suggesting benefits that extend beyond clinical anxiety to the everyday stress reactivity most people are dealing with.

The research case: cortisol directly

This is where the evidence becomes most directly relevant to this book. Several studies have now found that probiotic supplementation reduces cortisol levels specifically, not just anxiety symptoms.[3,4] A study in athletes — a population under significant physical and psychological stress — found that probiotic supplementation reduced cortisol and other stress biomarkers compared to placebo.[4] The mechanism appears to involve both improved cortisol clearance via a healthier gut and modulation of the HPA axis through the gut-brain connection.

The research case: OCD and rumination

One of the more intriguing areas of probiotic research involves obsessive-compulsive disorder and rumination — the repetitive, intrusive thought patterns that are a significant feature of anxiety and cortisol overload. Early research suggests that specific probiotic strains may reduce these patterns by modulating the gut-brain signaling involved in their production.[5] This is early-stage research, but it's consistent with the broader picture of the gut's involvement in anxiety pathology.

The research case: specific populations

Several studies have looked at probiotic effects in populations with elevated cortisol baselines. Pregnant women given probiotics showed reduced cortisol and improved mood outcomes.[6] Burnout patients given a multi-strain probiotic showed significant reductions in cortisol and improvements in energy and mood.[7] Workers under chronic workplace stress showed cortisol reductions and improved stress resilience with probiotic supplementation.[8] The pattern across these populations is consistent: probiotics help, and they help more in people whose cortisol is already elevated.

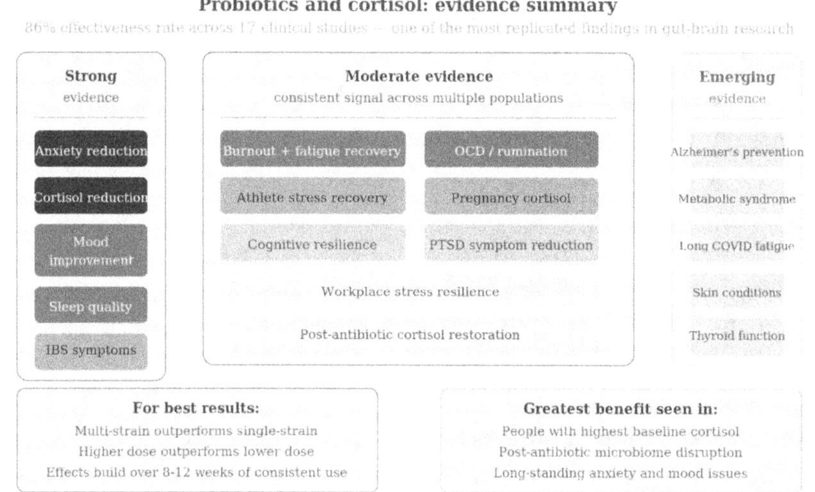

Fueling the gut reduces cortisol

Probiotics get most of the attention in gut-cortisol conversations, but probiotics are only as effective as the environment they're introduced into. A gut that's inflamed, nutrient-depleted, and running on processed food is a difficult environment for beneficial bacteria to establish and thrive in. The nutritional context matters as much as the probiotic itself.

Glutamine: the gut's primary fuel

The cells that line your gut — the ones responsible for selective permeability, for keeping the right things in and the wrong things out — use glutamine as their primary energy source. When glutamine is depleted, which happens readily under chronic stress, gut lining integrity suffers. The tight junctions that prevent unwanted molecules from crossing into the bloodstream become compromised. The result is the leaky gut that enables the food sensitivity cascade described earlier in this chapter.

Glutamine supplementation supports gut lining repair and has been shown to reduce intestinal permeability in clinical studies.[9] It's available in powder form — the most practical delivery method for gut repair purposes — and is generally well-tolerated. The one caveat: avoid if you have sensitivity to MSG, as glutamine converts to glutamate in the body, which can be problematic for sensitive individuals.

Fish oil for the gut

The omega-3 fatty acids in fish oil have direct anti-inflammatory effects on the gut lining, and multiple studies show that fish oil supplementation improves gut microbiome composition in addition to reducing systemic inflammation.[10] For the gut-cortisol connection specifically, fish oil's ability to reduce both gut inflammation and cortisol levels simultaneously makes it a particularly efficient tool — one supplement, two of the most important targets.

Zinc carnosine for gut lining repair

Zinc carnosine is a specific zinc compound that has shown particular effectiveness for gut lining repair and has been studied specifically for its ability to protect and restore the gut epithelium.[11] It's distinct from regular zinc supplementation in its targeted gut effects and is worth knowing about for anyone dealing with significant gut lining damage. Standard doses are 75mg twice daily with food.

Hormones to help hormones: DHEA

DHEA — dehydroepiandrosterone — is a hormone produced by the adrenal glands that sits at a fascinating intersection of the cortisol story. It's produced by the same glands that produce cortisol, it shares precursor molecules with cortisol, and it functions in many ways as a physiological counterbalance to cortisol's effects.

When cortisol is chronically elevated, **DHEA** tends to decline. The adrenal glands are essentially prioritizing cortisol production at the expense of DHEA, which makes metabolic sense from a survival standpoint but creates real problems over time. Low DHEA is associated with accelerated aging, reduced immune function, poor mood, low energy, and reduced resilience to stress — exactly the cluster of symptoms that chronically stressed people complain about and that don't fully respond to cortisol management alone.

The DUTCH hormone test — mentioned in Chapter 1 — measures both cortisol and DHEA, and the ratio between them is one of the more clinically informative values in the whole panel. A high cortisol-to-DHEA ratio indicates a stress response that has been running long enough and hard enough to compromise the body's counterbalancing mechanisms. This is the hormonal signature of what conventional medicine dismisses as adrenal fatigue and what this book more accurately calls cortisol resistance.

DHEA supplementation: what the research shows

DHEA is available as a supplement in the United States without prescription, at doses typically ranging from 5mg to 50mg daily. The research on DHEA supplementation is mixed in ways that reflect the hormone's complexity — it affects different systems differently, individual responses vary considerably, and the dose that helps one person may be unhelpful or mildly problematic for another.

That said, several consistent findings are worth knowing about. DHEA supplementation in older adults with low baseline levels improves well-being, energy, mood, and in some studies libido.[12] It appears to reduce cortisol's catabolic effects on muscle and bone. And in people with diagnosed adrenal insufficiency, DHEA supplementation is well-established as a meaningful quality-of-life intervention.

For people with stress-related DHEA depletion, the cautious approach is to test first — measure your DHEA-S level, which is the storage form of DHEA and more stable than DHEA itself — and supplement based on what the test shows rather than assuming you're deficient. Starting doses of 5–10mg daily are appropriate for most people new to DHEA supplementation, with increases based on response and retesting.

Work with a provider who understands hormone optimization when adding DHEA, particularly if you're already on other hormonal interventions. DHEA converts to both estrogen and testosterone in the body, and the balance of that conversion varies by individual. It's not complicated to manage, but it benefits from monitoring.

DHEA quick reference

- **What it is:** An adrenal hormone that counterbalances cortisol's effects
- **What low DHEA looks like:** Fatigue, low mood, poor stress resilience, reduced libido, accelerated aging markers
- **How to check it:** DHEA-S blood test (more stable than DHEA); optimal with DUTCH hormone panel
- **Supplementation:** 5–50 mg daily; start at 5–10 mg and adjust based on response
- **Cautions:** Converts to estrogen and testosterone — monitor levels; work with a provider for optimization

Chapter 8 summary

The gut and cortisol are not separate stories. They are the same story told from two directions. Chronic stress damages the gut; a damaged gut amplifies the cortisol response. The cortisol that rises in response to stress prevents the gut from healing; the gut that can't heal keeps cortisol elevated.

Breaking that cycle requires addressing both ends simultaneously — and the tools exist to do it. Probiotics to restore the microbiome. Berberine where overgrowth is contributing. MRT testing to identify and remove reactive foods. Glutamine, fish oil, and zinc carnosine to repair the gut lining. DHEA where the adrenal contribution to the cycle needs direct support.

None of these are dramatic interventions. None of them require a prescription. All of them have meaningful research behind them, and all of them are things I have used with real clients and seen real results from.

- *Fix the gut and watch how many other problems start to resolve.*

- References

1 Probiotic meta-analysis and anxiety. Nutrients. 2019. https://pmc.ncbi.nl m.nih.gov/articles/PMC6769995/

2 Probiotic RCT and psychological distress. Brain Behav Immun. 2015. https://pubmed.ncbi.nlm.nih.gov/25862297/

3 Probiotics and cortisol. Neurogastroenterol Motil. 2021. https://pubm ed.ncbi.nlm.nih.gov/33107152/

4 Probiotics in athletes and cortisol. J Int Soc Sports Nutr. 2019. https://p ubmed.ncbi.nlm.nih.gov/30791984/

5 Probiotics and OCD/rumination. Acta Neuropsychiatr. 2019. https://p ubmed.ncbi.nlm.nih.gov/30782253/

6 Probiotics in pregnancy and cortisol. J Nutr. 2018. https://pubmed.ncb

i.nlm.nih.gov/30321269/

7 Probiotics in burnout and cortisol. Nutrients. 2020. https://pubmed.nc bi.nlm.nih.gov/33207703/

8 Probiotics and workplace stress. Nutrients. 2019. https://pmc.ncbi.nlm .nih.gov/articles/PMC6769995/

9 Glutamine and intestinal permeability. Nutrients. 2021. https://pmc.nc bi.nlm.nih.gov/articles/PMC8000653/

10 Fish oil and gut microbiome. Nutrients. 2020. https://pmc.ncbi.nlm.n ih.gov/articles/PMC7510520/

11 Zinc carnosine and gut lining repair. J Gastroenterol. 2009. https://pu bmed.ncbi.nlm.nih.gov/19107356/

12 DHEA supplementation and well-being. J Clin Endocrinol Metab. 2006. https://pubmed.ncbi.nlm.nih.gov/16249270/

13 MRT food sensitivity testing. J Integr Med. 2008. https://www.david publisher.com/Public/uploads/Contribute/5aa87a8e491ec.pdf

14 Gut microbiome and cortisol metabolism. Neuroscience. 2020. https://pmc.ncbi.nlm.nih.gov/articles/PMC7442351/

15 Berberine and gut microbiome selectivity. Front Cell Infect Microbiol. 2021. https://pmc.ncbi.nlm.nih.gov/articles/PMC8477025/

16 Berberine and gut inflammation. Pharmacol Res. 2020. https://pubme d.ncbi.nlm.nih.gov/32001386/

17 Antibiotic effects on microbiome diversity. Nature. 2016. https://pub med.ncbi.nlm.nih.gov/27043005/

9

Chapter 9

MEAL PLANNING

Enough science. Let's eat.

Everything in the previous eight chapters has been building toward this: the practical reality of what you put on your plate, day after day, meal after meal. The science matters — I wouldn't have written eight chapters of it if it didn't. But science that doesn't translate to Tuesday dinner isn't doing you much good.

This chapter is the bridge. It takes everything we've covered — the gut-cortisol loop, the nutrient depletion cycles, the anti-inflammatory principles, the GABA-supporting foods, the probiotic-fermented food connection — and turns it into actual meals you can make in an actual kitchen, on a weeknight, without a culinary degree or a four-hour window.

The goal is not perfection. Cortisol management through food isn't about eating flawlessly — it's about building a default that's good enough consistently enough that your body has what it needs to regulate itself. One perfect meal a week surrounded by chaos doesn't move the needle. Seven decent meals — meals that include protein, healthy fat, fiber, fermented foods, and herbs wherever possible — absolutely does.

How to use this chapter

This chapter gives you three things: a set of guiding principles for cortisol-friendly eating (brief, because we've covered the science already), a one-week sample meal plan with cortisol-busting principles built into every meal, and a prep guide for making the week's eating manageable without spending your Sunday in the kitchen.

The meal plan is a template, not a prescription. Swap proteins, change vegetables based on what's available and in season, adjust quantities for your household size. The underlying structure is what matters: protein and healthy fat at every meal, a fermented food somewhere in the day, herbs and spices used freely, organic grains and legumes where possible, and the phone in another room while you eat.

Chapter 10 has the recipes referenced here. Each recipe is labeled with its primary cortisol-supporting benefit so you can swap in your own favorites that work through the same mechanisms.

The ten principles of cortisol-friendly eating

These are the distilled principles from Chapters 4, 5, and 8 — the practical version you can keep in your head without referring back to the science every time you open the refrigerator.

- **Protein at every meal.** Your body can't make hormones, neurotransmitters, or the gut lining without adequate protein. Aim for a palm-sized portion at breakfast, lunch, and dinner. Wild fish, pastured eggs, grass-fed meats, organic poultry, and whole-fat plain dairy are the most nutrient-dense sources.
- **Healthy fat with every meal.** Fat slows glucose absorption, prevents cortisol-triggering blood sugar spikes, and provides the raw material for steroid hormone production. Olive oil, avocado, eggs, fatty fish, nuts and seeds, and butter on your vegetables are not indulgences — they are

functional nutrition.

- **Fermented food daily.** Yogurt, kefir, sauerkraut, kimchi, kombucha, fermented vegetables — rotate through them. You don't need all of them every day. You need at least one, most days, consistently. These are your gut bacteria's direct delivery system.

- **Herbs and spices in everything.** This is the easiest upgrade most people aren't making. Rosemary, thyme, sage, turmeric, ginger, cardamom, mint, and lemon zest are not finishing touches — they are active ingredients. Use them liberally. They are GABA-supporting, anti-inflammatory, and cortisol-reducing, and they cost almost nothing.

- **Organic grains and legumes.** If you eat grains and legumes — and there's no reason you can't — choose organic to avoid glyphosate exposure. Glyphosate disrupts GABA and damages the gut lining. Organic oats, wild rice, quinoa, and properly prepared legumes are all cortisol-friendly carbohydrate sources.

- **Colorful vegetables at every meal.** Antioxidants from plants reduce the inflammatory signaling that keeps cortisol elevated. Dark leafy greens, beets, bell peppers, sweet potatoes, and cruciferous vegetables all contribute different antioxidant compounds. Variety is the point — try to eat several colors each day.

- **Front-load your calories.** Eating larger meals earlier in the day and tapering toward evening aligns with your cortisol rhythm — cortisol is naturally highest in the morning and lowest at night. Eating a big meal late at night disrupts this natural ebb, affects sleep quality, and tends to worsen morning cortisol. Eat dinner early when possible.

- **Bone broth as a weekly staple.** Bone broth provides glycine — the calming amino acid that also supports gut lining repair and sleep quality. It's easy to make in a slow cooker, available pre-made in most grocery stores, and one of the most nutrient-dense and affordable additions to a cortisol-busting kitchen.

- **Herbal tea in the evening.** This is one of the simplest and most underused cortisol tools available. A cup of chamomile, tulsi, passionflower, valerian, or lemon balm tea 30–60 minutes before bed is doing pharmacological work on your stress response while also creating a wind-down ritual that signals your nervous system that the day is over.

- **Put the phone away and eat.** The act of eating in a stressed, distracted state suppresses stomach acid, reduces digestive enzyme production, impairs nutrient absorption, and keeps your nervous system in fight-or-flight mode during a meal that was supposed to be a recovery opportunity. This is physiology, not etiquette. Set the phone down. Eat the food.

The cortisol plate

If you don't want to think about meal planning more than you have to, use this as your default framework for every meal:

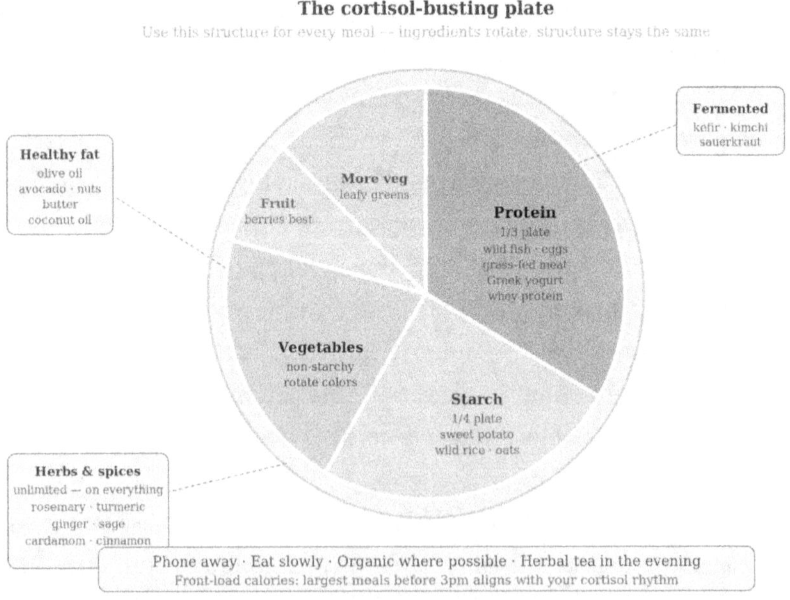

The cortisol plate diagram: Half the plate = non-starchy vegetables (dark leafy greens, cruciferous vegetables, colorful peppers, beets, zucchini). Quarter = high-quality protein (wild fish, pastured eggs, grass-fed meat, organic poultry). Quarter = complex carbohydrate (sweet potato, wild rice, quinoa, organic oats, sourdough). Plus: a healthy fat source on or alongside everything (olive oil, avocado, butter, nuts, full-fat dairy). Plus: a fermented food somewhere in the meal or day. Herbs and spices: unlimited, on everything.

The plate works as a template for any protein, any vegetable, any starch. Wild salmon with roasted sweet potato and wilted spinach. Organic chicken thighs with quinoa and steamed broccoli. Pastured eggs with sautéed greens and sourdough. The structure is always the same — the ingredients rotate based on what's seasonal, available, and within budget.

Meal timing for cortisol balance

Cortisol follows a natural daily rhythm — the cortisol awakening response peaks in the first 30–60 minutes after you wake up, then gradually declines through the day, reaching its lowest point in the hours before sleep. Eating in alignment with this rhythm — rather than against it — makes cortisol management considerably easier.

Morning: eat within an hour of waking

The morning cortisol spike is there for a reason: it mobilizes energy for the day ahead. If you skip breakfast or delay eating significantly, blood sugar drops, cortisol rises further to compensate, and you're starting the day with elevated stress hormones before anything stressful has even happened. A protein-and-fat-forward breakfast — eggs, yogurt, smoked salmon, or nut butter — stabilizes blood sugar and works with the natural cortisol rhythm rather than extending the spike unnecessarily. Personally, I don't do classical breakfast at all. For example, I open up a can of safe-catch tuna, mix it with walnut oil , vinegar, and salt, and put it on a bed of greens, sesame, and pumpkin seeds.

Midday: *the most important meal for sustained energy*

Lunch is where most people make their biggest cortisol-related dietary mistakes — skipping it entirely when busy, grabbing something processed and convenient, or eating at their desk while staring at a screen. All three approaches keep cortisol elevated through the afternoon. A proper lunch — protein, vegetables, healthy fat, eaten sitting down without a screen — produces a different afternoon than any of these alternatives. The difference in focus, mood, and 4pm energy is measurable within a week of making the change.

Afternoon: *manage the slump without cortisol spikes*

The 2–4pm energy dip is a natural circadian phenomenon and doesn't need to be fought with caffeine. A small snack with protein and fat — nuts, an egg, a small portion of yogurt — addresses it without the cortisol-stimulating effect of an additional coffee. Herbal teas with adaptogenic herbs like tulsi or ashwagandha are a better afternoon tool than coffee for people dealing with cortisol dysregulation.

Evening: *smaller, earlier, and herb-forward*

Eating late at night disrupts sleep quality and the natural nocturnal cortisol drop. Aim for dinner at least three hours before bed. Keep the evening meal lighter than lunch — this isn't about restriction, it's about letting your digestive system rest before sleep. Follow dinner with an herbal tea. This simple ritual — dinner, herbal tea, no more eating — has a measurable effect on sleep quality and morning cortisol that most people notice within the first week of consistent practice.

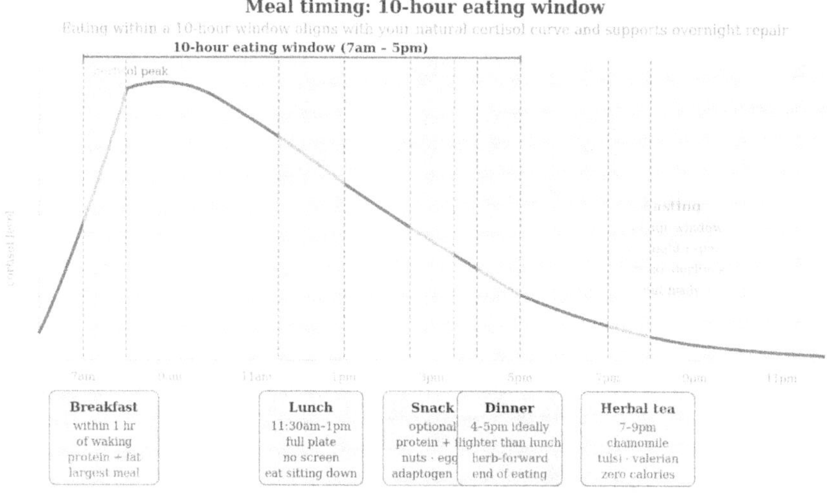

Sample one-week cortisol-busting meal plan

Below is a full week of cortisol-busting meals. Each day includes breakfast, lunch, dinner, and an evening snack or herbal tea. The week is designed to include: salmon at least twice, organ meats or bone broth at least twice, fermented food daily, herbs and spices in every meal, and a calming herbal tea each evening.

Recipes for starred items appear in Chapter 10. Everything else can be assembled without a formal recipe using the cortisol plate framework.

Day
Breakfast
Lunch
Dinner
Snack / herb tea

Monday
Scrambled eggs with arugula & rosemary, kefir with berries, green tea
Wild salmon salad, olive oil dressing, sauerkraut on the side, organic rye crispbread
Grass-fed beef stir-fry, bok choy, turmeric, ginger, wild rice
Brazil nuts, chamomile-tulsi tea

Tuesday
Overnight oats with chia seeds, cardamom, cinnamon, almond butter, kefir
Lentil & vegetable soup (organic), bone broth base, fresh rosemary, cheese
Baked organic chicken thighs, roasted sweet potato, green beans, lemon zest
Apple with almond butter, lemon balm tea

Wednesday
Smoked salmon on rice cake (or sourdough), avocado, capers, cucumber, matcha
Chicken bone broth with brown rice noodles, bok choy, soft-boiled egg, ginger
Grass-fed lamb chops, roasted beets, sauteed broccoli, garlic, olive oil
Pumpkin seeds, valerian or passionflower tea before bed

Thursday
Greek yogurt (whole-fat) with walnuts, honey, tulsi tea
Tuna & white bean salad, olive oil, celery, parsley, organic corn tortillas
Wild salmon with miso glaze, steamed broccoli, brown rice, sesame seeds
Wild blueberries, rose tea

Friday
Veggie omelette with goat cheese, sun-dried tomatoes, basil, fresh fruit
Turkey lettuce wraps, avocado, cucumber, kimchi, fresh mint
Grass-fed beef burger (skip the bun), roasted sweet potato wedges, mixed salad
Kefir smoothie with frozen berries, chamomile tea

Saturday
Full breakfast: pastured eggs, bacon, sautéed mushrooms

Homemade bone broth soup, roasted vegetable medley, fermented pickles

Whole roasted organic chicken, root vegetables, fresh sage, garlic

Mixed nuts, jujube, evening tea

Sunday

Shakshuka (eggs in tomato-herb sauce), rice cake (or sourdough), plain kefir, fresh herbs

Leftover roasted chicken, large salad, olive oil vinaigrette, kombucha

Pan-seared wild cod, lemon-caper sauce, roasted asparagus, wild rice pilaf

Nut butter on celery sticks, tulsi-rose tea

The Sunday prep guide

The biggest barrier to eating this way consistently isn't motivation — it's friction. When you come home exhausted at 6:30pm and there's nothing ready, the path of least resistance is whatever can be ordered or microwaved. Removing that friction requires about 90 minutes on Sunday. Here's how to spend them:

Sunday prep: 90 minutes for a calmer week

START (15 min): Start the slow cooker

Put a whole chicken carcass or beef bones in the slow cooker with water, apple cider vinegar, onion, garlic, salt, and herbs. Set to low. It will cook all day and produce bone broth for the week. If you're using store-bought broth, skip this.

PROTEINS (20 min): Cook your week's proteins

Hard-boil a batch of eggs (8–10). Bake or poach 2–3 chicken breasts or thighs with herbs. Leave salmon and other fish for the day you're cooking them fresh — fish doesn't hold as well as chicken.

GRAINS (15 min hands-off): Cook a big batch

One pot of wild rice, quinoa, or organic oats takes 20–30 minutes of mostly hands-off time and will cover multiple lunches and dinners. Cook it while you do other things.

VEGETABLES (20 min): Roast a big tray

Chop whatever vegetables need using up — sweet potatoes, beets, broccoli, cauliflower, bell peppers, zucchini — toss with olive oil and herbs, roast at 400°F for 25–30 minutes. Roasted vegetables last 4–5 days in the refrigerator and improve almost every meal they're added to.

FERMENTS (5 min): Set out, don't prepare

Make sure you have sauerkraut or kimchi in the refrigerator, kefir or yogurt available for breakfast, and a bottle of kombucha or two. These don't need prep — they just need to be there.

HERBS AND TEAS (5 min): Organize for the week

Set out your evening tea collection in a visible spot — not buried in the cupboard. Visible is accessible. Put your supplement bottles somewhere equally visible. Default behavior goes toward what requires no decision.

The batch cooking formula

Batch cooking doesn't require elaborate meal prep or identical lunches every day. It requires one protein, one grain, one roasted vegetable, and one sauce or dressing — all interchangeable. Here's the formula:

- **1 cooked protein:** rotisserie chicken, hard-boiled eggs, baked salmon, or cooked ground beef
- **1 cooked grain:** wild rice, quinoa, organic oats, or sourdough for toast
- **1 roasted vegetable:** whatever is seasonal — usually 2–3 different vegetables on one tray
- **1 raw salad base:** mixed greens, arugula, or chopped romaine that holds

well in the refrigerator
- **1 dressing or sauce:** a simple olive oil and lemon vinaigrette, a tahini sauce, or a miso-ginger dressing
- **1 fermented food:** sauerkraut, kimchi, kefir, or plain yogurt

From these six components you can assemble a different meal every day of the week with five minutes of effort. Grain bowl with chicken, roasted vegetables, and tahini sauce. Salad with salmon, avocado, and vinaigrette. Eggs over rice with kimchi. Chicken in lettuce wraps with miso dressing. The combinations are endless; the prep is done once.

Eating this way on a budget

I hear this concern often, and it's legitimate. Quality protein and organic produce do cost more than processed food. But the gap is smaller than it was five years ago, and there are ways to make cortisol-friendly eating work at almost any budget:

- **Canned wild salmon and sardines** are among the most nutrient-dense, affordable proteins available. The omega-3 content is equivalent to fresh fish at a fraction of the cost.
- **Eggs** remain one of the best nutritional values in any grocery store. Pastured eggs cost more than conventional; the difference in omega-3 content, vitamin D, and choline is significant.
- **Organic frozen vegetables** are nutritionally equivalent to fresh and considerably cheaper. Frozen spinach, broccoli, edamame, and mixed vegetables are reliable pantry staples.
- **Buy organic for the Dirty Dozen** (highest pesticide load: strawberries, spinach, kale, peaches, pears, nectarines, apples, grapes, bell peppers, cherries, blueberries, green beans) and conventional for the Clean Fifteen (lowest pesticide load: avocados, sweet corn, pineapple, onions,

papaya, asparagus, frozen peas, kiwi, cabbage, mushrooms, mangoes, sweet potatoes, watermelon, carrots, cauliflower).

- **Grow herbs.** A small pot of rosemary, mint, and basil on a windowsill produces fresh herbs continuously for months. The cortisol-reducing aromatics alone make this worthwhile.
- **Make your own bone broth.** A chicken carcass that would otherwise be discarded produces 2–3 liters of mineral-rich broth in a slow cooker. It costs essentially nothing and lasts a week in the refrigerator.

You don't have to eat perfectly to eat well. Good enough, consistently, is better than perfect occasionally.

The ritual of eating well

Everything in this chapter is about food as medicine. But food is also culture, connection, pleasure, and one of the few moments in a day when you can genuinely stop and be present. The cortisol-friendly meal is not just the one with the right macros — it's the one eaten slowly, at a table, without a screen, with attention to how the food tastes and smells and feels.

The ritual of preparing food is itself cortisol-reducing. The chopping, the smelling of herbs cooking in olive oil, the steam rising from a pot of bone broth — these sensory experiences activate the parasympathetic nervous system in ways that are measurable and meaningful. Cooking is not a chore to be optimized away. It is a recovery activity that your nervous system was designed to benefit from.

If you take one thing from this chapter beyond the meal plan, let it be this: eat more slowly, with more attention, more often than you currently do. The food matters. How you eat it matters nearly as much.

10

Chapter 10

CHAPTER 10

RECIPES

These are some of my favorite recipes that I love to make myself. They can help you manage cortisol and stress. Keep in mind that if you are sensitive or allergic to any of these foods, make sure to substitute ingredients where needed.

Each recipe carries a benefit label:

- Anti-inflammatory — reduces the inflammation-cortisol loop
- GABA-supporting — herbs and foods that calm the nervous system
- Gut-healing — fermented foods, bone broth, and gut-lining support
- Adrenal-nourishing — replenishes nutrients that cortisol depletes
- Blood sugar-balancing — prevents the cortisol spike that follows a glucose crash

Swap proteins, vegetables, and grains freely. The structure is what creates the cortisol benefit.

Teas & drinks

Soothing London Fog

● **GABA-supporting** • **Anti-inflammatory** • Serves 1 • 8 min

Any tea that has lavender becomes a special drink. This is a super simple cortisol-busting tea you can enjoy any time of the day.

INGREDIENTS

- Boiling water
- Decaf Earl Grey tea leaves
- Lavender buds or 1 drop food-grade lavender essential oil
- Raw coconut butter or heavy whipping cream
- Honey, to taste

DIRECTIONS

1. Add tea leaves and lavender buds to a tea diffuser. Pour boiling water over and steep 3–5 minutes.
2. Mix in desired amount of coconut butter and honey. Alternatively, add a small drop of food-grade lavender essential oil in place of the buds.

Heidi's note: Lavender is one of the most clinically documented cortisol-reducing herbs in this book — one study showed a 70% cortisol reduction from lavender aromatherapy alone. Breathing the steam from this cup counts.

Chamomile Matcha Tea

● **GABA-supporting** • **Blood sugar-balancing** • Serves 1 • 10 min

Making your own matcha drink lets you control quality and skip the presweetened sugar that indirectly creates cortisol imbalance. Adding chamomile helps dampen cortisol and adds a pleasant earthiness.

INGREDIENTS

- 1 tsp organic matcha powder
- 12 oz boiling water
- 1 tsp organic chamomile buds or 1 chamomile tea bag
- Whipping cream or coconut butter (optional)

DIRECTIONS

1. Add boiling water to your mug. Whisk in matcha with a frother.

2. Using a tea infuser, add chamomile buds and steep 5 minutes, or use a tea bag and remove after 5 minutes.

3. Mix in coconut butter or cream if desired.

Heidi's note: *Organic matcha delivers L-theanine, which balances the caffeine and reduces anxiety. Chamomile adds immediate cortisol-lowering effects. If green tea makes you jittery, address your COMT gene first with magnesium and P5P (see Chapter 7).*

Tulsi Turmeric Tea

● **Anti-inflammatory** • **Adrenal-nourishing** • Serves 1 • 10 min

Tulsi is an all-time favorite of mine because it is both relaxing and energizing. You can also buy turmeric tulsi tea bags at health food stores.

INGREDIENTS

- 1 tsp loose tulsi leaves
- ½ tsp turmeric
- 1 tbsp raw coconut butter or heavy whipping cream
- Pinch of black pepper
- 10–12 oz boiling water
- 1 tsp honey (optional)

DIRECTIONS

1. Boil water. Infuse tulsi leaves, turmeric, and black pepper in a tea infuser for at least 5 minutes.

2. Remove infuser. Stir in coconut butter and honey. Serve.

Heidi's note: *Tulsi manages stress, reduces blood pressure, and improves immune function — with no major side effects across 24 clinical studies. The black pepper enhances turmeric absorption by 2,000%. Don't skip it.*

Relaxing Lavender-Honey Hot Cocoa

⬤ **GABA-supporting • Anti-inflammatory** • Serves 1 • 8 min

This recipe was born after a shortened night of sleep. Lavender and chamomile help the body adapt to stress, and this drink perks me up in a way no cup of coffee can.

INGREDIENTS

- 12 oz boiling water
- 2 tsp cacao powder or cocoa powder
- 1 tsp raw honey
- 1 tsp vanilla extract
- 1 tsp chamomile buds or lavender buds
- 1 tbsp raw coconut butter or heavy whipping cream

DIRECTIONS

1. Add boiling water to your mug.

2. Using a metal tea infuser, steep the lavender or chamomile buds.

3. Add remaining ingredients and stir until honey and coconut butter are completely melted.

Adaptogen Kefir Smoothie

● **Gut-healing** • **Adrenal-nourishing** • Serves 1 • 5 min
INGREDIENTS

- 250ml plain whole-fat kefir
- 1 cup frozen mixed berries
- 1 banana (frozen for creaminess)
- 1 tbsp almond butter
- 1 tsp ashwagandha powder (optional)
- 1 tsp ground flaxseed
- Drizzle of honey to taste

DIRECTIONS

Blend all ingredients until smooth. Taste and adjust honey. Serve immediately.

Heidi's note: Kefir provides more probiotic strains than yogurt plus meaningful protein. Ashwagandha reduces cortisol by up to 30% in clinical research. Berries deliver antioxidants that protect against cortisol-related oxidative damage.

Smoothies

Mixed Berry Smoothie

● **Anti-inflammatory** • **Blood sugar-balancing** • Serves 1 • 5 min
Avoid protein powders with artificial ingredients like sucralose — they sneak into many brands and negate the health benefits.

INGREDIENTS

- 1 cup raspberries, blueberries, or strawberries (or a mix; frozen works)
- ½ tsp Ceylon cinnamon
- ½ cup celery, cut into 1–2 inch pieces

- 1 cup milk
- 1 cup ice (omit if using frozen berries)
- 1 scoop unflavored or natural vanilla whey protein powder (20–30g protein)

DIRECTIONS

Blend all ingredients until smooth.

Heidi's note: *Celery in a smoothie delivers apigenin, magnesium, and 3-n-butylphthalide — all nerve-supportive. Ceylon cinnamon (not cassia) stabilizes blood sugar without coumarin concerns. Berries provide antioxidants that blunt cortisol-related oxidative damage.*

Citrus-Ginger Smoothie

● **Anti-inflammatory** • **Gut-healing** • Serves 2 • 5 min

This keeps me going all morning and into the afternoon. Citrus helps bind hormonal toxins in the gut. Greek yogurt can make this tart — feel free to omit if you prefer a more subtle flavor.

INGREDIENTS

- 1 cup filtered water
- 1 tsp orange zest
- 1 fresh orange, peeled
- ½ cup celery, cut into 2-inch pieces
- Juice of 1 lime or lemon
- 2 packets natural stevia (omit if using stevia-sweetened powder)
- 2 tsp fresh ginger, grated
- ½ tsp ground cardamom or Ceylon cinnamon
- 1 cup plain Greek yogurt
- 1 scoop natural grass-fed whey vanilla protein powder
- 1 tsp Lion's Mane mushroom powder (optional)
- Ice, if desired

DIRECTIONS

Combine all ingredients in a blender, blend about 1 minute, and serve.

Heidi's note: *Orange zest delivers limonene, which supports GABA function. Cardamom reduces cortisol in an 8-study meta-analysis. Lion's Mane adds cortisol-reducing and nerve-growth-factor benefits. This smoothie is doing remarkable cortisol work while tasting like sunshine.*

Breakfasts

Herb and Cheese Omelet

● **GABA-supporting** • **Adrenal-nourishing** • Serves 1 • 10 min

INGREDIENTS

- 3 eggs
- ¼ cup whole milk or half and half
- 1 tbsp chopped fresh chives
- 1 tbsp fresh rosemary or 1 tsp dried rosemary (or herbs of choice)
- Salt and pepper to taste
- ½ tbsp butter
- 3 tbsp Swiss cheese, grated
- 1 tbsp parmesan cheese, grated

DIRECTIONS

1. Whip eggs with milk, chives, rosemary, salt, and pepper until all white is incorporated.

2. Melt butter over high heat in a 10" nonstick skillet until bubbly.

3. Pour in egg mixture, pulling toward center from each side.

4. Remove from heat when eggs no longer run but are still quite moist. Add cheese to the top half, fold, then invert onto a plate. Rest 1 minute before serving.

Heidi's note: *Rosemary in eggs sounds unusual and tastes remarkable. The* *rosmarinic acid in rosemary enhances GABA and counters cortisol. Eggs provide choline, vitamin D, and the fat-soluble vitamins depleted by chronic stress.*

Protein-Boosted Scrambled Eggs

● **Adrenal-nourishing** • **Blood sugar-balancing** • Serves 1–2 • 7 min
INGREDIENTS

- 4 large eggs
- ½ cup 2% cottage cheese (organic or Daisy brand)
- ⅛ tsp Himalayan salt
- Large pinch of your favorite herbs or herbal blend
- Freshly ground black pepper
- Extra-virgin olive oil

DIRECTIONS
1. Whisk eggs, cottage cheese, salt, herbs, and pepper in a bowl.
2. Heat a ceramic nonstick skillet over medium-low. Drizzle with oil. Pour in eggs.
3. Slowly scrape toward center with a spatula as the bottom sets, creating soft folds, about 2 minutes. Serve with fresh fruit if desired.

Heidi's note: Adding cottage cheese more than doubles the protein per serving without changing the texture noticeably. Higher protein breakfast = more stable blood sugar = less cortisol reactivity through the morning.

Easy Egg Muffins

● **Adrenal-nourishing** • **Blood sugar-balancing** • Serves 3–4 • 30 min
Make a batch and freeze for easy weekday breakfasts.
INGREDIENTS

- 9 large pasture-raised eggs
- ½ cup whole-milk organic cottage cheese
- 1 tsp cumin seed, coarsely ground
- 2 tsp dried oregano
- ½ tsp Himalayan salt, ¼ tsp pepper
- 1½ cups chopped vegetables (olives, bell peppers, onions, mushrooms, broccoli, or arugula)
- 1 cup grated sharp cheddar cheese
- Extra-virgin olive oil for greasing

DIRECTIONS

1. Preheat oven to 375°F. Grease a ceramic muffin tin liberally with olive oil.

2. Place 2 tbsp vegetables into each muffin tin.

3. Blend eggs, cottage cheese, salt, and pepper in a blender about 30 seconds until smooth.

4. Pour egg mixture into muffin wells, filling almost to the top.

5. Bake 18 minutes, until centers no longer look wet and edges are barely golden. Do not overcook.

26. Cool in tin, loosen gently with a knife, remove. Finish cooling on a wire rack.

Tip: Freeze extras. Reheat from frozen at 350°F for 12 minutes.

Cottage Cheese Breakfast Bowl

● **Gut-healing** • **Adrenal-nourishing** • Serves 1 • 5 min
INGREDIENTS

- 1 cup cottage cheese — no-additive brand (organic or Daisy brand)
- ½ cup fresh pineapple or berries (frozen works well too)
- 1 tsp fresh basil or ½ tsp fresh thyme (dried works too)

DIRECTIONS

Arrange all ingredients in a bowl and serve.

Heidi's note: Fresh basil contains apigenin and rosmarinic acid. Pineapple adds bromelain, an anti-inflammatory enzyme. This is as simple as breakfast gets and as nutritionally complete.

All-Natural Protein Yogurt Parfait

● **Gut-healing** • **Anti-inflammatory** • Serves 1 • 2 min

I like a small amount of maple syrup here to cut the tartness of plain yogurt — this way you control the carbohydrates while getting antioxidants that maple syrup provides.

INGREDIENTS

- 1 cup plain yogurt
- ¼ cup walnuts, hemp seeds, or other nuts
- ½ cup berries or banana (frozen berries work)
- Small drizzle of real maple syrup (optional)

DIRECTIONS

Layer all ingredients into a bowl and serve.

Heidi's note: Walnuts contain omega-3s, magnesium, and melatonin — yes, walnuts contain melatonin. Berries deliver antioxidants. Real maple syrup contains manganese and zinc; it is not nutritionally equivalent to corn syrup.

Savory Low-Carb Chickpea Pancakes

● **Blood sugar-balancing** • **Anti-inflammatory** • Serves 2 • 40 min (incl. soaking)

A versatile recipe from a chef friend. Adapt the spice to suit whatever you are serving alongside it.

INGREDIENTS

- 1 cup chickpea flour
- 1 cup water
- ½ tsp turmeric
- 2 tbsp minced vegetables such as onion and green pepper (or minced apple for sweet versions)
- Olive oil to coat the pan

DIRECTIONS

1. Mix all ingredients. Allow to sit 30 minutes to hydrate the chickpea flour.

2. Heat olive oil in a ceramic skillet over medium heat.

3. Cook each pancake until golden brown on each side, about 3–4 minutes per side.

Tip: Use cinnamon if serving with fruit; use Italian seasoning and garlic if serving with a savory dish. Pairs beautifully with eggs and fresh greens.

Salads & lighter meals

Tuna Lettuce Wraps

● **Anti-inflammatory** • **Blood sugar-balancing** • Serves 2 • 10 min
INGREDIENTS

- 1 (4-oz) can light tuna — not Albacore (high mercury)
- 2 tbsp avocado mayonnaise
- 1 tsp Dijon mustard
- 1 tbsp diced onions
- ½ tsp cumin or fennel seeds
- ½ cup shredded carrots
- ½ avocado, sliced

- 8 romaine lettuce leaves

DIRECTIONS

4. Combine all ingredients except avocado in a bowl and stir until mixed.

5. Spread mixture over lettuce leaves and top with avocado slices.

6. Roll up as you would a wrap and serve.

Heidi's note: Fennel seeds are a GABA-enhancing spice frequently overlooked in cortisol conversations. Avocado mayonnaise uses avocado oil instead of inflammatory seed oils. Light tuna is preferable to Albacore for regular consumption.

Refreshing Shrimp Salad

● **Anti-inflammatory • Adrenal-nourishing** • Serves 2 • 5 min

My go-to recipe on hot summer days. Shrimp provides astaxanthin for brain and eye health — light, refreshing, and satisfying all at the same time.

INGREDIENTS

- 2 cans salad shrimp, drained
- 1 tsp lemon zest
- Juice of 1 lemon
- 2 tbsp olive oil
- 2 tbsp sweet onion, diced
- ¼ cup celery, diced
- 1 tsp dried dill
- 4 cups leafy green salad mix or romaine lettuce, chopped

DIRECTIONS

1. Combine all ingredients except leafy greens in a bowl.

2. Serve over lettuce.

Heidi's note: Shrimp contains astaxanthin, one of the most potent antioxidants in any food, with documented neuroprotective and cortisol-protective effects. It also provides iodine, zinc, and selenium — critical for adrenal and thyroid function.

Savory and Sweet Broccoli Salad

● **Anti-inflammatory** • **Blood sugar-balancing** • Serves 6 • 10 min
INGREDIENTS

- 5 cups broccoli, chopped into bite-size pieces
- ½ cup sweet onion, chopped
- ⅛ cup roasted almonds
- ¼ cup raisins or dried cherries
- Dressing: 3 tbsp olive oil, 2 tbsp apple cider vinegar, 2 tbsp maple syrup, 1 tbsp Dijon mustard, 1 tsp dried sage, ¼ tsp salt, ½ tsp pepper

DIRECTIONS

1. Combine broccoli, onion, almonds, and raisins in a bowl.
2. Whisk all dressing ingredients together.
3. Pour dressing over vegetables and stir to combine. Improves with several hours of marinating.

Heidi's note: Sage in the dressing contributes memory-supporting and cortisol-reducing compounds. Broccoli provides sulforaphane, one of the most potent anti-inflammatory compounds in any vegetable. Apple cider vinegar stabilizes blood sugar.

Dressed Up Sardines

● **Adrenal-nourishing** • **Anti-inflammatory** • Serves 1 • 5 min
Sardines are so healthy and delicious — using flavored ones is the key to trying them. They are one of the most sustainable fish and rich in hormone-healthy omega-3 fatty acids.

INGREDIENTS

- 1 can sardines (lemon-seasoned works well here)
- 2 cups leafy greens

- Chopped carrots, broccoli, bell peppers
- 1–2 tbsp chopped pistachios or almonds
- 1 orange, cut into bite-sized pieces
- Lemon dressing: ¼ cup fresh lemon juice, ¼–⅛ cup extra-virgin olive oil, 1 tsp Dijon mustard, ½ tsp garlic powder, ¼ tsp sea salt, ½ tsp maple syrup, ½ tsp thyme, ½ tsp dill

DIRECTIONS

1. Whisk all dressing ingredients together.
2. Toss sardines into lettuce and vegetable mixture. Dress generously.
3. Add pistachios and orange slices.

Heidi's note: *Canned sardines are the most affordable and nutrient-dense omega-3 source available. They contain calcium, vitamin D, B12, selenium, and zinc — a comprehensive adrenal restoration in a can. See thehealthyrd.com/best-s ardines-in-a-can for choosing quality brands.*

Seared Tuna Poke Bowl

● **Anti-inflammatory • Blood sugar-balancing** • Serves 2 • 30 min

INGREDIENTS

- 8–12 oz raw ahi tuna, cubed
- Marinade: 4 tbsp green onions; 1 tsp tamari; ¾ tsp sesame oil; ¼ tsp ginger, minced; ¼ tsp sriracha
- Cauliflower rice: 3 cups riced cauliflower; 2½ tsp olive oil; ½ tsp sesame oil; sea salt
- Bowls: ⅞ cup cucumber; 1 avocado, cubed; sesame seeds; sliced nori
- Sauce: 1½ tbsp avocado mayonnaise + ½ tbsp sriracha

DIRECTIONS

1. Combine tuna marinade, cover tuna, and chill at least 10 minutes.
2. Heat skillet on medium-high. Add 1 tbsp oil. Sear tuna 1–1½ min per

side for medium-rare. Slice into ½-inch slices.

3. For cauliflower rice: heat oils in a large skillet. When smoking, add cauliflower and sauté until golden, about 10 minutes. Season with salt.

4. Divide rice between bowls. Add tuna, cucumber, avocado. Garnish. Drizzle with mayo-sriracha.

Heidi's note: *Cauliflower rice significantly reduces the glycaemic load while adding glucosinolates that support liver cortisol metabolism. Ahi tuna provides protein and omega-3s. This bowl is doing a lot of cortisol work in a beautiful package.*

Soups

Hot and Sour Soup

● **Gut-healing** • **Anti-inflammatory** • Serves 6–8 • 20 min

Like restaurant hot and sour soup but more satisfying because of the much higher protein content.

INGREDIENTS

- 8 cups chicken or beef bone broth
- 8 oz shiitake or baby bella mushrooms, thinly sliced
- 2 (8-oz) cans bamboo shoots, drained (optional)
- 1 thinly sliced onion
- ¼ cup rice vinegar, or more to taste
- ¼ cup tamari sauce
- 2 tsp chili garlic sauce
- ¼ cup cornstarch
- 6 large eggs, whisked
- 3 pounds sliced chicken thighs, pork, or steak
- 4 green onions, thinly sliced
- White or black pepper

DIRECTIONS

1. Set aside ¼ cup broth. Add remaining broth, mushrooms, bamboo shoots, protein, vinegar, tamari, and chili garlic sauce to a stockpot. Heat to a simmer.

2. Whisk reserved broth with cornstarch until smooth. Once simmering, stir in and cook 1 minute until thickened.

3. Stir in half the green onions. Season with salt and pepper.

4. Stir soup in a circle and drizzle in whisked eggs in a thin stream to create egg ribbons.

5. Serve immediately, garnished with remaining green onions.

Heidi's note: *Shiitake mushrooms contain lentinan, an immune-enhancing compound, and eritadenine for cardiovascular health. Bone broth base provides glycine. The protein load from eggs and meat supplies the amino acids depleted by chronic stress.*

Relaxing Chicken and Wild Rice Soup

● **Gut-healing** • **Adrenal-nourishing** • Serves 8 • 40 min

Nothing beats chicken soup for easing cortisol. This version uses antioxidant-rich wild rice instead of processed noodles.

INGREDIENTS

- 4 large stalks celery
- 1 sweet onion
- 1 pound carrots (about 4 medium)
- 2 tbsp extra-virgin olive oil
- 2 bay leaves
- 2 tsp dried rosemary, crushed
- 1½ tsp dried sage or 1 tbsp fresh sage, minced
- 3 large cloves garlic
- 1½ pounds chicken breasts, skinned and boned
- 1 lemon, zested and juiced

- 8 cups chicken bone broth
- 1 cup wild rice
- 2 tsp Himalayan salt, pepper to taste

DIRECTIONS

1. Slice celery and carrots ½ inch. Chop onion.

2. Sweat vegetables with olive oil, rosemary, and sage on medium-low for about 10 minutes with lid on. Add garlic and salt during the last 2 minutes.

3. Cut chicken into bite-sized pieces. Turn heat high, add chicken and broth, bring to a boil. Reduce and simmer 10 minutes.

4. Add wild rice and cook 30–45 minutes to desired texture.

5. Add lemon juice and zest. Season with salt and pepper.

Heidi's note: *Rosemary and sage together deliver rosmarinic acid in every bowl. Lemon zest provides limonene. Wild rice has significantly higher antioxidants and a lower glycaemic index than processed pasta. This soup tastes like genuine care.*

Main dishes

Pistachio-Crusted Chicken with Cauliflower-Leek Mash

● **Adrenal-nourishing** • **Blood sugar-balancing** • Serves 4 • 40 min
INGREDIENTS

- 4 chicken breasts
- Crust: ½ cup pistachios, finely chopped; 1 tsp dried oregano; ½ tsp cumin; ½ tsp salt
- Mash: 1 head cauliflower; 2 leeks; 1 scoop collagen powder; salt to taste

DIRECTIONS

1. The mash: Boil cauliflower and leeks in salted water until very soft. Drain, then mash with collagen powder and salt until creamy.

2. The crust: mix pistachios with oregano, cumin, and salt.

3. Press pistachio crust firmly onto chicken breasts.

4. Bake at 375°F for 25–30 minutes until crust is toasted and chicken is cooked through.

5. Serve over the cauliflower-leek mash.

Heidi's note: *Pistachios are unusually high in B6, which supports COMT enzyme activity, GABA production, and green tea catechin processing. Collagen in the mash provides glycine for gut lining and sleep support. Cauliflower supports liver cortisol metabolism.*

Spiced Beef & Cauliflower with Sweet Potato

● **Anti-inflammatory** • **Adrenal-nourishing** • Serves 4 • 1 hr 15 min

A vibrant, aromatic dish inspired by Middle Eastern flavors, with tender beef and roasted cauliflower and sweet potatoes.

INGREDIENTS

- 1 lb beef, cubed
- 1 tsp salt
- 2 cups cauliflower florets
- 2 cups diced sweet potatoes
- 1 onion, sliced
- Spices: 1 tsp cardamom, 1 tsp turmeric, 1 tsp ginger, ½ tsp nutmeg, 1 tsp cumin
- 2 tbsp coconut oil
- ½ can coconut milk
- 1–2 cups water

DIRECTIONS

1. Heat 2 tbsp coconut oil in a large pot. Brown beef on all sides, then add onion and cook until softened.

2. Stir in all spices and salt. Cook on low 1 hour with 1–2 cups water and coconut milk.

3. Toss cauliflower with coconut oil, salt, and turmeric. Roast at 425°F until golden and tender, about 20–25 minutes. Roast sweet potatoes alongside.

4. Serve beef over or alongside roasted vegetables.

Heidi's note: *Cardamom, turmeric, ginger, and cumin together create a powerful anti-inflammatory and cortisol-reducing spice combination with overlapping clinical evidence. Grass-fed beef provides zinc, iron, and B12. Coconut milk adds lauric acid with antimicrobial gut benefits.*

Easy Coconut Chicken

● **Gut-healing** • **Anti-inflammatory** • Serves 4–6 • 55 min

A family favorite — both savory and rich while healing for the gut and the mind.

INGREDIENTS

- 2 lb chicken thighs or breasts, bone-in if possible
- 1 sweet onion, sliced
- 1 clove garlic, minced
- 1 tbsp dried oregano
- 1 tbsp dried sage
- ½ tbsp ghee or extra-virgin olive oil
- 2 cups canned coconut milk
- ½ cup chicken bone broth
- 1 tsp salt, ½ tsp pepper

DIRECTIONS

1. Sauté onion and garlic in ghee in a cast iron skillet on medium until softened, about 3 minutes.

2. Add chicken and brown for about 12 minutes, flipping halfway.

3. Season with oregano, sage, salt, and pepper.

4. Add coconut milk and bone broth; bring to a simmering boil. Deglaze

the pan.

5. Reduce heat to low and simmer 35 minutes until tender. Check every 10 minutes to prevent sticking.

Heidi's note: Sage is the standout herb here — it reduces cortisol and improves both short- and long-term memory in clinical research. Bone broth base provides glycine. Coconut milk adds lauric acid and fat-soluble vitamins that support hormone production.

Simplified Butter Chicken

● **Anti-inflammatory** • **Adrenal-nourishing** • Serves 6–8 • 25 min

A comforting family favorite that my family thinks is better than most restaurants. Use whole coriander and cumin seeds crushed with a mortar and pestle to release the flavors.

INGREDIENTS

- 2 lb chicken thighs, boneless, skinless
- 3 tbsp butter + 4 tbsp butter (added at end)
- 1 medium sweet onion, diced
- 3–4 cloves garlic, minced
- 2 inches fresh ginger, grated
- Spices: 2 tbsp garam masala, 1 tbsp curry powder, 1 tsp turmeric, 1 tsp paprika, 1 tbsp cumin (crushed), 1 tbsp coriander (crushed)
- 1 tsp salt, ½ tsp black pepper
- 15 oz can tomato sauce
- ½ cup heavy cream
- ½ cup fresh cilantro, chopped
- Shirataki rice or cauliflower rice for serving

DIRECTIONS

1. Heat butter in a large skillet over medium heat. Add onion, cook 5 minutes. Add garlic and ginger, cook 5 more minutes. Season with salt and

pepper.

2. Stir in all spices and cook until fragrant, about 1 minute.

3. Add tomato sauce and cream. Bring to a boil, cook 5 minutes until slightly thickened.

4. Add chicken and cook through, about 15–20 minutes.

5. Finish with remaining 4 tbsp butter. Serve over shirataki or cauliflower rice, top with cilantro.

Heidi's note: *Freshly crushed whole cumin and coriander seeds release volatile compounds that pre-ground spices have largely lost. All four main spices — garam masala, turmeric, cumin, coriander — have documented anti-inflammatory effects. This is the spice combination that makes the meal.*

Wild Salmon Salad

● **Anti-inflammatory** • **Adrenal-nourishing** • Serves 4 • 15 min

For a super healthy and refreshing meal, this is a favorite. You can also use your favorite herbs and spices.

INGREDIENTS

- 1½ pounds wild salmon fillets
- 4 tbsp extra-virgin olive oil, divided
- 1 cup sweet onion, finely diced and divided
- ½ tsp paprika
- 1 tsp fennel seed
- 2 tsp Worcestershire sauce
- 1 tsp dill weed
- 4 tbsp lemon juice plus lemon wedges
- 12 cups mixed greens and other vegetables
- ½ cup celery, sliced
- Salt and pepper to taste

DIRECTIONS

1. Drain fish on paper towels. Heat 1 tsp oil in a skillet over medium-high.

2. Add onion and fennel and stir-fry. When onion begins to brown, add fillets over onions. Brush top of each fillet with 2 tsp oil. Sprinkle with paprika, dill, and salt.

3. When pan-side is opaque, about 3 minutes, turn fish. Splash with Worcestershire sauce and lemon juice. Cover and reduce heat to low for 2 minutes. Remove from heat.

4. Prepare salad: arrange greens and remaining onion and celery on plates. Drizzle with remaining olive oil and lemon juice.

5. When ready to serve, turn fish over and roughly flake over the lettuce. Serve at room temperature with lemon wedges.

Heidi's note: *Wild salmon eaten twice weekly is one of the most evidence-backed dietary interventions for reducing baseline cortisol. Fennel seed enhances GABA. Dill contains apigenin. This recipe is elegant enough for guests and easy enough for Tuesday.*

Sheet Pan Lemon Salmon, Potatoes & Green Beans

● **Anti-inflammatory** • **Blood sugar-balancing** • Serves 4 • 30 min
INGREDIENTS

- 1 (24-oz) package baby Yukon Gold potatoes, cut in small cubes
- 3 tbsp extra-virgin olive oil, divided
- 1 tsp salt; ¾ tsp pepper
- 2 tbsp lemon juice
- 4 small cloves garlic, finely chopped
- 1 tbsp chopped fresh dill, plus more for garnish
- 4 (5-oz) wild salmon fillets
- 1 (8-oz) package trimmed thin green beans

DIRECTIONS

1. Preheat oven to 400°F. Line a large rimmed baking sheet with

parchment.

2. Toss all ingredients together on the pan.

3. Cook 20–25 minutes until done.

Tip: One pan, one cleanup. Dill provides apigenin. Garlic provides allicin, an antimicrobial that supports gut health.

Slow-Cooker Swiss Steak

● **Adrenal-nourishing • Anti-inflammatory** • Serves 4 • 3 hrs 30 min
I grew up eating this delicious meal, so I want to share it with you.
INGREDIENTS

- 2 lb beef sirloin or round steak, cut into 2-inch strips
- ¾ tsp garlic powder
- 3 tbsp olive oil
- ¼ cup beef broth + 1 tbsp cornstarch
- ½ cup chopped onion
- 2 large green bell peppers, roughly chopped
- 1 (14.5-oz) can stewed tomatoes with liquid
- 2 tbsp coconut aminos
- 1 tbsp fresh rosemary, chopped (or 1 tsp dried)
- 1 tsp honey

DIRECTIONS

1. Sprinkle beef with garlic powder. Sear in oil about 5 minutes per side. Transfer to slow cooker.

2. Mix broth and cornstarch until dissolved. Pour over beef.

3. Add onion, peppers, tomatoes, coconut aminos, rosemary, and honey.

4. Cook on High 3–4 hours or Low 6–8 hours.

Heidi's note: Slow cooking extracts collagen from the beef, converting to gelatin that supports gut lining integrity. Rosemary adds rosmarinic acid. Bell peppers provide vitamin C — one of the nutrients most rapidly depleted by cortisol. This dinner essentially makes itself.

Slow-Cooker Cuban Mojo Roast Pork

● **Adrenal-nourishing** • **Anti-inflammatory** • Serves 4–6 • 8 hrs (mostly hands-off)

INGREDIENTS

- 4–6 lb bone-in or boneless pork shoulder
- 8 cloves garlic
- ½ medium Spanish or yellow onion
- 1 tbsp dried oregano
- 1 tsp ground cumin
- ½ tsp kosher salt, ½ tsp black pepper
- 1 cup orange juice
- ½ cup lime juice

DIRECTIONS

1. Smash garlic. Slice onion. Mix oregano, salt, cumin, and pepper.

2. Pat pork dry. Cut 8 large slits 1–2 inches deep. Stuff a garlic clove into each slit.

3. Place in slow cooker. Pour citrus juices over, rubbing into slits. Coat with spice mixture. Top with onion. Refrigerate 8 hours or overnight, flipping once.

4. Cook on LOW about 8 hours until fork-tender.

5. Transfer to baking sheet. Rest 5–10 minutes. Tear into large chunks. Spoon cooking liquid over top. Broil 5–10 minutes until browned and crisp.

6. Serve with lime wedges, rice, and black beans.

Heidi's note: The orange and lime marinade delivers limonene. Cumin and oregano add rosmarinic acid. The cooking liquid is essentially a cortisol-busting broth worth saving for other uses.

Comforting Italian Meatloaf

● **Adrenal-nourishing** • **Anti-inflammatory** • Serves 6–8 • 1 hr 20 min

I've made this for over 20 years and my family devours it. I often make an extra and freeze it.

INGREDIENTS

- 3 pounds grass-fed ground beef
- 1 tsp salt
- 2 tbsp coconut flour or ½ cup breadcrumbs
- 3 tbsp dried parsley
- 2 tbsp dried oregano or Italian seasoning
- 2 eggs
- 1 cup marinara sauce, divided, plus extra for topping
- 1 tbsp garlic powder
- ½ cup parmesan cheese

DIRECTIONS

1. Preheat oven to 325°F. Cover a baking sheet with foil or parchment.

2. Combine all ingredients except ½ cup of the marinara in a large bowl. Mix thoroughly with hands.

3. Shape into a rectangle about 1½ inches thick, 6 inches wide, 10 inches long. Top with remaining marinara.

4. Bake about 60 minutes until cooked through. Rest 10 minutes before slicing.

Heidi's note: *Grass-fed beef contains 2–5x more omega-3s and significantly higher CLA than grain-fed, plus more zinc and iron. Parsley is rich in apigenin. Oregano provides rosmarinic acid. This is comfort food that is doing cortisol work.*

Saffron Cod

● **Anti-inflammatory • Adrenal-nourishing** • Serves 4 • 10 min
INGREDIENTS

- 1 pinch saffron (about ⅛ tsp)
- 1½ lb cod or tilapia, cut into ¼–¾ inch fillets
- Salt and pepper to taste
- ¾ tsp turmeric
- ¼ cup gluten-free flour
- ¼ cup olive oil
- 3 tbsp lemon juice
- 1 lemon, cut into wedges

DIRECTIONS

1. Grind saffron and bloom in 2 tbsp hot water. Set aside.
2. Dry fish on both sides. Season with salt and pepper.
3. Mix turmeric and flour. Dredge fish and shake off excess.
4. Heat oil in skillet over medium-high until hot.
5. Add 2 tbsp lemon juice to the saffron water.
6. Add fish to pan — it should sizzle immediately. Cook 2 minutes until golden and crispy.
7. Flip, pour lemon-saffron mixture over fish, cook second side 2 minutes. Serve with lemon wedges.

Heidi's note: Saffron at 30 mg daily reduces depression symptoms comparably to SSRIs in five clinical trials. This recipe delivers a meaningful per-serving dose. Combined with anti-inflammatory turmeric and omega-3s from wild cod, this is one of the most pharmacologically active recipes in the book.

Shirataki Noodle Chicken Stir-Fry

● **Blood sugar-balancing** • **Anti-inflammatory** • Serves 2–4 • 40 min

Shirataki (Miracle or Konjac) noodles have zero calories, are gluten-free and low-carb. When I first tried them, I was surprised at how tasty they were.

INGREDIENTS

- 1 (14-oz) package shirataki noodles
- Sauce: 1½ tbsp tamari or coconut aminos; 1½ tbsp toasted sesame oil; 1½ tsp honey; 1 tsp chili paste (optional)
- Avocado or olive oil for the pan
- 1 cup grated carrots
- 1 cup pea sprouts
- 1 tsp garlic, grated; 1 tsp ginger, grated
- ¾ cup cilantro leaves
- 2 cups cooked chicken, shredded
- ½ cup scallions, thinly sliced
- 1½ tsp black sesame seeds, toasted

DIRECTIONS

1. Pour noodles into a colander and rinse with cold water. Add to saucepan with enough water to cover. Bring to a boil, reduce to low, simmer 15 minutes. Drain, rinse, return to pan.
2. Mix sauce ingredients and pour over noodles. Toss gently, cover, and set aside.
3. Coat a sauté pan with oil on medium heat. Add carrots, sprouts, garlic, ginger. Sauté until carrots are tender, about 5 minutes.
4. Add cilantro, chicken, scallions, and sesame seeds. Stir 30 seconds. Turn off heat.
5. Add noodles to the pan on low. Toss gently until everything is warm. Serve.

Heidi's note: *Shirataki noodles are made from konjac root — essentially a prebiotic fiber that feeds beneficial gut bacteria without raising blood sugar. An excellent low-cortisol substitute for blood-sugar-spiking noodles. Ginger and garlic add anti-inflammatory compounds throughout.*

Stuffed Mushrooms

● **Gut-healing** • **GABA-supporting** • Serves 4 • 30 min

A great low-carb appetizer rich in antioxidants and probiotics from the goat cheese.

INGREDIENTS

- 4 oz chevère goat cheese, softened
- 3 tbsp olive oil
- 8 large button mushrooms
- 2 cloves garlic
- ¼ cup sweet onion
- ½ tsp dried rosemary and/or thyme
- ⅛ tsp paprika
- 1 tsp lemon zest (optional)

DIRECTIONS

1,Preheat oven to 425°F. Mince garlic. Finely chop mushroom stems and onion.

2. Combine goat cheese, 2 tbsp olive oil, garlic, paprika, and lemon zest in a bowl. Set aside.

3. Sauté onion and mushroom stems in remaining oil until slightly browned, about 5 minutes. Add rosemary or thyme. Mix into cheese mixture.

4. Spoon mixture into mushroom caps, heaping above them. Bake about 20 minutes until bubbly and browned.

Heidi's note: *Goat cheese is more easily digested than cow's milk cheese and* *contains probiotics. Mushrooms provide ergothioneine, an antioxidant amino acid unique to fungi with neuroprotective effects. Rosemary and thyme deliver GABA-supporting rosmarinic acid.*

Sheet Pan Sausage and Vegetables

● **Anti-inflammatory** • **Blood sugar-balancing** • Serves 4 • 25 min

Sheet pan dinners are the best way to quickly get a healthy meal on the table.

INGREDIENTS

- 1–2 packs all-natural chicken or beef sausage, sliced
- 2 cups broccoli florets, bite-sized
- 2 cups carrots, sliced
- 1 cup onions, bite-sized pieces
- 1 cup mushrooms, sliced
- 1 tbsp dried oregano or assorted herbs
- 1 tsp fennel seeds
- Olive oil for drizzling

DIRECTIONS

1. Preheat oven to 400°F. Cover a sheet pan with parchment.
2. Place all ingredients on pan. Drizzle with olive oil and toss to combine.
3. Cook 20 minutes or until vegetables and sausage are slightly browned.

Tip: Choose sausages with simple ingredient lists: meat, spices, salt. Avoid fillers, corn syrup, or carrageenan.

Treats

Blueberry-Lavender Frozen Yogurt

● **Gut-healing** • **GABA-supporting** • Serves 2–4 • 5 min + 2–4 hrs freezing

A favorite of mine for an indulgent treat free of preservatives and processed sugars. Lavender buds give this an extra hormonal-balancing effect and are absolutely delicious here.

INGREDIENTS

- 1 cup plain whole-milk yogurt
- ¾ cup wild blueberries (or any berry; frozen works fine)
- 1 tbsp raw honey
- 1 tsp lavender buds

DIRECTIONS

1. In a bowl, mix berries, honey, and lavender buds together, mashing with a spoon until juices are released.

2. Stir in plain yogurt. Adjust honey if desired.

3. Serve fresh or freeze 2–4 hours. Works beautifully in a Ninja Creami on the Lite ice cream setting.

Heidi's note: Wild blueberries have among the highest antioxidant content of any fruit. Lavender buds deliver linalool and GABA-active compounds internally, not just through aromatherapy. Whole-milk yogurt provides protein, fat-soluble vitamins, and probiotics. This is genuinely dessert that works for you.

A note on cooking as cortisol medicine

The act of cooking — the chopping, the smell of herbs heating in olive oil, the steam rising from a pot, the sensory engagement of making something with your hands — activates the parasympathetic nervous system in ways that are measurable and meaningful. Cooking is a recovery activity. It is one of the oldest forms of stress management available, and it happens to produce the exact nutrients your body needs to regulate the stress response more effectively.

The recipes in this chapter are not magic. They are the application of everything in this book to real food, made in a real kitchen, on a real Tuesday evening. That's enough. That's the whole point.

11

Chapter 11

CONCLUSION

THE WHOLE WORLD COULD USE LESS CORTISOL

I think about the clients who come to me depleted.

Not just nutritionally — though that is almost always part of the picture. Depleted in the way that a person gets when they have been carrying too much for too long without the right tools, the right support, or even the right information. They arrive at my office having done everything right by conventional medicine's standards, and still feeling like themselves has become someone they only vaguely remember.

This book is for them. And it is for you.

Excess cortisol and hormonal imbalances don't have to control your health and your life. While modern lifestyles and societal pressures are constantly driving our bodies into a state of imbalance, nurturing ourselves can go a long way to keeping you from the ravages of these stressors. This takes a multi-pronged approach: prioritizing sleep, guided meditation, nutritious foods, replacing nutrients that stress depletes, and balancing inflammation with healing herbs and spices.

What I hope you take from this book is not a protocol. It is a framework. Cortisol is the organizing principle — the thread that runs through your gut health, your hormonal balance, your mood, your weight, your sleep, your resilience. When you understand that, the individual tools stop feeling like an overwhelming list of things to do and start feeling like pieces of a coherent whole. The supplements, the herbs, the meal planning, the probiotics, the DHEA conversation — all of them are working toward the same thing. Giving your body what it needs to regulate itself.

When in doubt, heal your gut and provide your body with natural anti-inflammatory medicinal foods, herbs, and supplements.

Nature's wide array of healing compounds are put on this earth to give our bodies checks and balances in this complex hormonal system that we have. Using ancestral wisdom dovetailed with clinical research is the best way to go. The herbs in Chapter 7 have been used by cultures across centuries and continents. The modern research is not discovering these things — it is confirming what careful human observation has known for a long time.

But you should always stay curious and keep learning. This is just a starting point. There is so much out there to discover. To keep the process going, I highly encourage you to seek out information at its source: the National Library of Medicine, available at PubMed. While there is a lot of medical jargon in there, you can still glean powerful healing tools from the research. It can also arm you with the evidence that your healthcare providers want. Don't hesitate to go to your appointments prepared. After all, they are stressed to the max themselves — most providers are required to see 30 patients a day. New research is happening all of the time but your provider doesn't have the time to access it. Your providers don't have time to get into the details of your health unless you advocate for yourself.

If you suspect you are sensitive to foods, do food sensitivity testing as described in Chapter 8. If your cortisol symptoms aren't shifting despite doing everything else right, the gut is almost always the missing piece. If the gut is already addressed and symptoms persist, look at your hormonal picture — DHEA, progesterone, thyroid — and work with a practitioner who can help you optimize the whole system rather than manage individual symptoms.

A note on healing as a ripple effect

Here is something I have watched happen over and over in 26 years of clinical practice: when one person in a household starts to feel better, the people around them start to feel better too. Not immediately, not automatically, but through the quiet transmission of changed habits, changed moods, changed food, changed conversations. Healing is contagious in the best possible way.

The whole world could use less cortisol, more love, and more information. You now have all three.

I would be honored if you share this book with your friends and your loved ones. When one person heals, it starts a ripple effect. Go cause some trouble.

With gratitude,
Heidi Moretti, MS, RD, CLT

12

Chapter 12

GLOSSARY

Terms appear in bold sage green at their first appearance in the main text. This glossary provides definitions for all highlighted terms.

ACE inhibitors: A class of blood pressure medications used primarily to treat high blood pressure, heart failure, and certain types of kidney disease. They work by blocking the angiotensin-converting enzyme (ACE), preventing the narrowing of blood vessels and elevation in blood pressure.

Acid reflux: A condition in which stomach acid or stomach contents flow back up into the esophagus.

Acupuncture: A form of Traditional Chinese Medicine (TCM) in which thin needles are inserted into the body to promote healing.

Adaptogens: Natural substances, including herbs, roots, mushrooms, or plant extracts that help the body resist and adapt to various stressors, including physical, emotional, environmental, and chemical exposures.

Adrenal fatigue: A term used to describe a collection of symptoms including chronic fatigue, body aches, digestive issues, sleep disturbances, and cravings for salt or sugar. It is a result of prolonged stress. More accurately described as cortisol resistance in clinical literature.

Adrenal response: The body's reaction to stress, primarily stemming from the adrenal glands.

Agonist: A substance that activates cell receptors, often mimicking the action of natural substances like neurotransmitters or hormones in the body.

Anti-inflammatory: Any compound or action that prevents or counteracts inflammation.

Antioxidants: Substances that reduce oxidative stress in the body.

Aromatherapy: The therapeutic use of essential oils, derived from plants, to improve physical, emotional, and spiritual well-being.

Aromatic oils: Fragrant oils, typically derived from plants, that possess a distinct and pleasant smell and have a direct effect on the limbic system of the brain.

BDNF (Brain-Derived Neurotrophic Factor): A protein essential for the growth and function of neurons in the brain and nervous system. BDNF helps optimize nerve health, learning, memory, and emotional regulation and promotes the development of new neurons.

Body dysmorphia: A mental health condition in which a person spends a lot of time worrying about perceived flaws in their appearance.

B vitamins: A group of eight essential water-soluble vitamins known as the B-complex vitamins. These nutrients play primary roles in cellular metabolism, energy production, red blood cell formation, muscle health, brain health, and nervous system function.

Butyrate: A short-chain fatty acid produced by beneficial gut bacteria during fermentation of dietary fiber. It serves as the primary fuel for cells lining the gut and helps maintain the integrity of the gut lining.

COMT gene (Catechol-O-methyltransferase gene): Also referred to as the worrier/warrior gene, provides instructions for producing the COMT enzyme, which breaks down compounds in the body, including neurotransmitters like dopamine, norepinephrine, and epinephrine. This gene regulation is crucial for maintaining balance in mood, stress response, focus, memory, and emotional control.

Cortisol burnout: An unbalanced cortisol response in your body, causing cortisol levels to be high at inappropriate times. It also causes the body to respond inappropriately to cortisol.

Cortisol resistance: A phenomenon in which cortisol stays chronically elevated and the body's receptors essentially stop responding to it properly. The signal keeps firing but nothing responds effectively. Analogous to insulin resistance.

Cortisone: The kinder, gentler version of cortisol for your body, converted from cortisol primarily in the liver, gut, kidneys, and fat tissue. To achieve ideal health, your cortisol-to-cortisone ratio should be low.

Cortisol/cortisone ratio: A biomarker that reflects the balance between the active glucocorticoid hormone cortisol and its inactive metabolite cortisone. A high ratio indicates chronic stress or impaired cortisol metabolism.

CoQ10 (Coenzyme Q10): A naturally occurring antioxidant compound found in the mitochondria of cells, essential for energy production and protection against oxidative stress.

DHEA (Dehydroepiandrosterone): A hormone produced by the adrenal glands that serves as a parent to other sex hormones including testosterone, progesterone, and estrogen. Chronically elevated cortisol tends to deplete DHEA over time.

DUTCH hormone test (Dried Urine Test for Comprehensive Hormones): A hormone test that measures estrogen, progesterone, testosterone, cortisol, DHEA-S, melatonin, and hormone metabolites. It captures daily hormonal fluctuations and metabolic activity, offering deeper insights than single-point blood tests.

EEG (electroencephalogram): A noninvasive test that records the electrical activity of the brain.

EMDR (Eye Movement Desensitization and Reprocessing): A structured psychotherapy designed to help individuals heal from trauma and distressing life experiences. Most widely used for PTSD but also effective for anxiety, depression, and other conditions linked to unresolved traumatic memories.

Enteric nervous system: The extensive network of neurons lining the gastrointestinal tract, sometimes called the "second brain," responsible for managing digestive function and communicating bidirectionally with the central nervous system.

Estrogen dominance: A type of hormonal imbalance where estrogen levels are relatively high compared to progesterone, even if estrogen levels are within the normal range. Associated with breast cancer risk, weight gain, and mood changes.

Fatty liver disease: A condition where excess fat builds up in the liver, also called Metabolic Associated Steatotic Liver Disease (MASLD). Closely linked to excess processed foods, obesity, insulin resistance, type 2 diabetes, and high blood pressure. Impairs cortisol-to-cortisone conversion.

Fight or flight: An intense physiological reaction in the body that occurs in response to a perceived threat or danger. Mediated primarily by the release of cortisol and adrenaline.

Flavone: A class of crystalline flavonoids, usually a natural yellow pigment, found in citrus fruits, celery, and other foods. Apigenin is a well-studied flavone with GABA-enhancing and cortisol-reducing properties.

Functional medicine: A patient-centered, science-based approach to healthcare that focuses on identifying and addressing the root causes of illness. This form of medicine views the body and mind as an integrated system and considers genetic, environmental, and lifestyle factors that influence long-term health and disease.

GABA (gamma-aminobutyric acid): The primary inhibitory neuro-transmitter in the brain and spinal cord that balances nerve signals, helping calm neural activity and maintain balance between excitatory and relaxing signals in the central nervous system. Cortisol dysregulation impairs GABA function; many cortisol-reducing herbs work by enhancing it.

Ghrelin: A hormone produced by gut endocrine cells in the stomach, sometimes called the "hunger hormone" because it increases the desire to eat. Elevated by chronic stress and poor sleep.

GLP-1 (Glucagon-Like Peptide-1): A naturally occurring hormone made in the intestines in response to eating that helps regulate blood sugar, appetite, and digestion. Also the basis of a class of prescription weight-loss and diabetes medications.

Glufosinate: An herbicide used widely in agriculture that has replaced some glyphosate use as legal pressure around glyphosate has grown. Carries similar concerns about gut and hormonal disruption.

Glyphosate: The active ingredient in the herbicide Roundup, sprayed on most conventionally grown wheat, corn, soy, oats, and legumes. Disrupts GABA function, damages the gut lining, and drives inflammation. Subject to over 100,000 legal claims and billions in settlements.

Gut-brain axis: A bidirectional communication network between the brain and the gut that uses nerve signals, hormones, and immune messengers. The vagus nerve is its primary highway. The state of the gut directly influences brain function, mood, and stress response.

Gut health: The overall state and function of the gastrointestinal tract, including the integrity of the gut lining, the balance of the gut microbiome, and the health of digestion and nutrient absorption.

Gut microbiome: A large community of trillions of microorganisms in the gut consisting primarily of bacteria, but also viruses, fungi, and archaea, that live mostly in the large intestine. Directly involved in cortisol regulation, serotonin production, immune function, and mental health.

Heart rate variability (HRV): A measure of the variation in time between consecutive heartbeats. A higher HRV can indicate better stress resilience and recovery, while a lower variability can be indicative of stress, fatigue, illness, or overtraining.

Hypnotherapy: A form of mental health therapy that uses hypnosis to promote a state of deep focus and openness to suggestion. Not a magical trance but a form of concentrated attention that works directly with the subconscious to change deeply rooted patterns. One of the most effective cortisol management tools available.

HPA axis (Hypothalamic-pituitary-adrenal axis): The body system that regulates stress and maintains the body's balance between the hypothalamus, pituitary gland, and adrenal glands. The master control system for cortisol production.

IBS (Irritable bowel syndrome): A type of chronic functional gastrointestinal disorder with symptoms of abdominal pain, bloating, and changes in bowel habits. Often linked to food sensitivities, an altered microbiome, and elevated cortisol.

Inflammation: A natural part of the body's reaction to injury and infection. When chronic — related to foods, toxins, or chemicals — it drives cortisol elevation and contributes to virtually all modern chronic diseases.

Leptin: A hormone made by fat cells that regulates long-term calorie balance in the body. Dysregulated by chronic cortisol elevation, contributing to difficulty losing weight.

Limbic system: A group of brain structures located deep within the brain that plays a central role in regulating emotions, motivation, memory, and behaviors essential for survival. The primary emotional processing center and a key regulator of the stress response.

Linoleic acid: An omega-6 fatty acid found abundantly in seed oils (soybean, canola, corn, sunflower). Excessive intake is pro-inflammatory and has been linked to increased inflammatory disease risk.

L-theanine: An amino acid found naturally in green tea that promotes calm focus by enhancing GABA activity without causing sedation. Balances the stimulating effects of caffeine.

Mediator Release Test (MRT): A food sensitivity test that measures the actual release of inflammatory mediators from white blood cells in response to 176 foods and food chemicals. More clinically accurate than IgG testing, which measures antibody exposure rather than inflammatory response.

Melatonin: A hormone in your body made in response to circadian rhythms of daylight and dark. Plays a role in sleep regulation. Produced partly in the gut and affected by cortisol dysregulation.

Microplastics: Small plastic particles that are insoluble in water, persistent in the environment, and found in oceans, soil, air, food, and human tissues. Directly impair the conversion of cortisol to cortisone, worsening the cortisol-to-cortisone ratio.

Mitochondrial: Relating to the mitochondria, the energy-producing structures within cells. SSRIs may impair mitochondrial function, which may contribute to their association with weight gain.

Neuro Linguistic Programming (NLP): An approach to communication, personal development, and psychotherapy that asserts a connection between neurological processes, language, and acquired behavioral patterns, and that these can be changed to achieve specific goals.

Nutraceutical: A term used to describe any product derived from food sources that provides health benefits beyond basic nutrition.

Parasympathetic nervous system: One of the three divisions of the autonomic nervous system that promotes relaxation — the "rest and digest" state. The target of most effective cortisol management interventions.

Probiotics: Live microorganisms that provide a health benefit when consumed in adequate amounts. Directly reduce cortisol, reduce anxiety, and improve gut microbiome composition. Multi-strain formulations at higher doses consistently outperform single-strain products.

Progesterone: A steroid hormone produced primarily in the ovaries, also by the adrenal glands. Low progesterone is associated with elevated cortisol and increased anxiety. Declining progesterone in perimenopause and menopause is linked to worsening cortisol patterns.

Proton pump inhibitors (PPIs): A class of medications that cause a strong and prolonged reduction in stomach acid by irreversibly inhibiting stomach acid production. Significantly impair nutrient absorption, disrupt gut bacteria, and are associated with increased risk of anxiety and depression.

PTSD (Post-traumatic stress disorder): A condition which impairs daily living that can develop after experiencing or witnessing a traumatic event involving actual or threatened death, serious injury, or sexual violence. Strongly associated with cortisol dysregulation and generational transmission.

REM sleep (Rapid Eye Movement): The stage of sleep most closely related to vivid dreaming, memory consolidation, and emotional regulation. Disrupted by caffeine even when sleep onset and duration appear normal.

Serotonin: A neurotransmitter with a wide range of functions in both the central nervous system and body tissues. Approximately 95% of the body's serotonin is produced in the gut. Supports mood, memory, reward, and gut motility. Directly suppressed by elevated cortisol.

SSRIs (Selective Serotonin Reuptake Inhibitors): A class of antidepressant medications that work by blocking the reabsorption of serotonin in the brain. Associated with weight gain in approximately half of users and potential mitochondrial effects with long-term use. Natural alternatives including saffron have shown comparable efficacy in multiple clinical trials.

Stress hormone: Refers primarily to cortisol, produced by the adrenal glands in response to stress. Also encompasses adrenaline (epinephrine) for acute stress responses.

Sympathetic nervous system: A division of the autonomic nervous system responsible for preparing the body for stress or emergency situations. The "fight or flight" state. Chronically activated in modern life.

Traditional Chinese Medicine (TCM): An alternative form of medicine rooted in ancient Chinese philosophy developed over thousands of years. Encompasses acupuncture, herbal medicine, cupping, therapeutic massage, qigong, and tai chi.

Transgenerational trauma: The phenomenon by which the effects of trauma are transmitted across generations, affecting the psychological and physiological health of descendants who did not directly experience the original trauma.

Vagus nerve: The longest and most complex of the 12 pairs of cranial nerves, originating in the brainstem and extending to the digestive tract, heart, and lungs. The primary highway of the gut-brain axis. Responsible for parasympathetic nervous system regulation and directly involved in cortisol management.

WHO (World Health Organization): A specialized agency of the United Nations responsible for international public health that sets health standards and provides leadership on health polic

13

Chapter 13

INDEX

Page numbers refer to book page numbers. Bold page numbers indicate primary discussion. Italicized page numbers indicate a diagram or table.

B

C

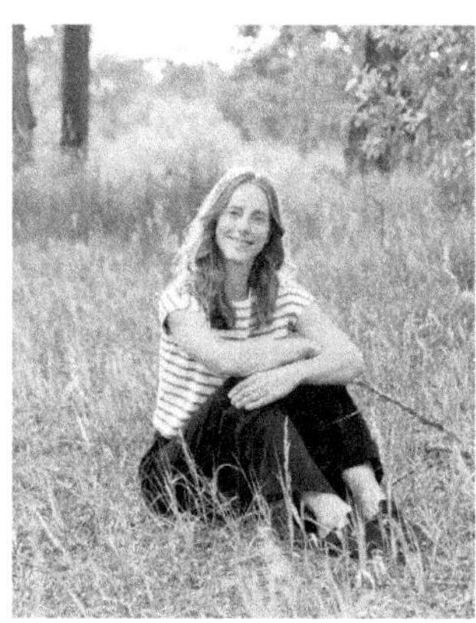

About the Author

Heidi Moretti, MS, RD, CLT, is a registered dietitian, author, LEAP practitioner, and owner of The Healthy RD LLC, a functional nutrition private practice, blog, and resource for people looking to find natural and scientifically proven remedies for health issues. She received postgraduate training through the Institute for Functional Medicine and is constantly using the National Library of Medicine to uncover natural medicine research.

She is the author of the bestselling books *Period Fix, Gut Fix, The Whole Body Guide to Gut Health*, and *The Elimination Diet Journal*. She has published numerous clinical research studies as principal investigator, including:

"Vitamin D3 repletion versus placebo as adjunctive treatment of heart failure patient quality of life and hormonal indices: a randomized, double-blind, placebo-controlled trial."

"Biotin Deficiency as a target for treating restless legs syndrome in chronic dialysis patients."

"Effects of protein supplementation in chronic hemodialysis and peritoneal dialysis patients."

"Prevalence of low albumin, suboptimal energy, and muscle stores in Asian dialysis patients."

Additionally, she worked for over twenty years at Providence Saint Patrick Hospital in Missoula, Montana, where she honed her clinical skills and continued to find ways to integrate functional medicine into a conventional world.

Heidi writes about nutrition, herbs, gut health, and cortisol management at thehealthyrd.com.

You can connect with me on:

◉ https://thehealthyrd.com

🐦 https://x.com/HeidiHmoretti

 https://www.facebook.com/thehealthyrd

Subscribe to my newsletter:

✉ https://thehealthyrd.com

Also by Heidi Moretti

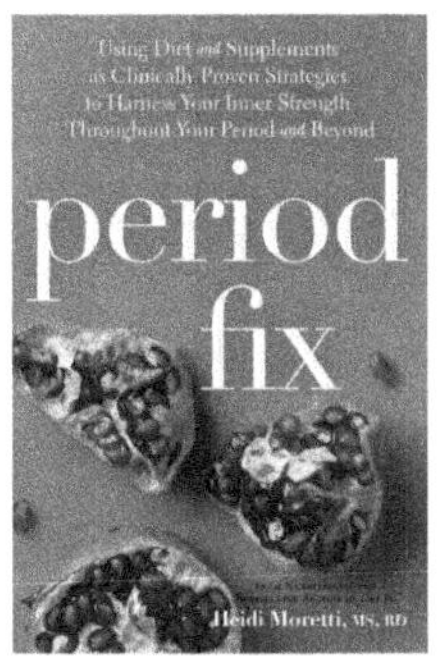

Period Fix

Women's period health is often relegated when it comes to research dollars and attention by doctors. Even worse, conventional medicine can end up making women feel worse instead of better! But there are many more options for optimizing your menstrual health than you may know and many of these start with food, nutrients, and safe herbal supplements as natural medicine.

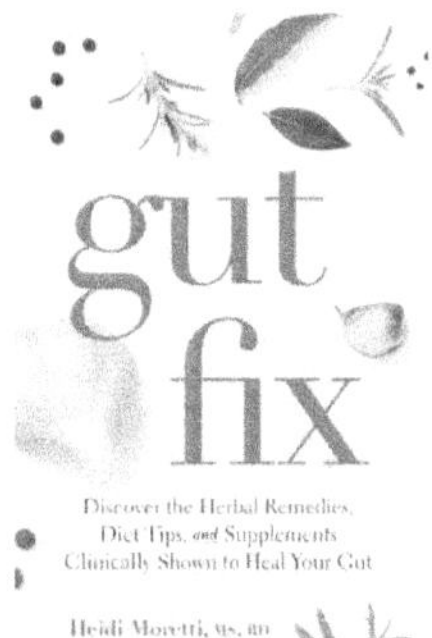

Gut Fix

Discouraged by visit after visit with your doctor about your gut issues, you feel like there is nowhere else to turn. But you haven't lost hope and you know that there has to be something out there that is safe and worth trying to help you feel better. That's where the Gut Fix book comes in. You are meant to feel better because the body heals when you give it what it needs. You want to use a natural approach to being free of heartburn and other gut conditions too but don't know where to start.